THE
LAUGHTER
EFFECT

T0363295

THE LAUGHTER EFFECT

How to Build Joy, Resilience and Positivity in Your Life

ROS BEN-MOSHE

NERO

Published by Nero,
an imprint of Schwartz Books Pty Ltd
22–24 Northumberland Street
Collingwood VIC 3066, Australia
enquiries@blackincbooks.com
www.blackincbooks.com

Copyright © Ros Ben-Moshe 2023
Ros Ben-Moshe asserts her right to be known as the author of this work.

ALL RIGHTS RESERVED.
No part of this publication may be reproduced, stored in a retrieval system,
or transmitted in any form by any means electronic, mechanical, photocopying,
recording or otherwise without the prior consent of the publishers.

9781760643331 (paperback)
9781743822852 (ebook)

 A catalogue record for this
book is available from the
National Library of Australia

Cover design by Tristan Main
Cover image: George Peters / iStock
Image on p.130: Clare Snow / Flickr
Text design by Marilyn de Castro
Typesetting by Typography Studio

Printed in Australia by McPherson's Printing Group.

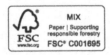

Contents

From the moment I picked up your book until I laid down, I was convulsed with laughter. Someday I intend reading it.

—Groucho Marx

To my dearly beloved parents, Bridget and Cyril,
for giving me the gift of life and laughter

Introduction

What soap is to the body, laughter is to the soul

—Yiddish proverb

We've all heard the saying that 'laughter is the best medicine'. But is it really that simple? Can a certain amount of laughter be the cure-all for a range of modern-day ailments, including loneliness and depression? What if you're not in the mood for laughing? Or perhaps you don't think you're especially funny, and your nearest and dearest aren't exactly a bag of laughs either. How, then, can you access this wellspring?

The good news is that if you're hesitant about channelling your inner comedian, or in the thick of a stressful situation, you can call on what I have coined the 'Laughter Effect'. This body-mind philosophy and practice based on science – with fundamentals dating to biblical times and ancient civilisations – is not, surprisingly, dependent on a joke or a funny situation. Rather, it's a holistic humour- and non-humour-based skillset that doesn't leave feeling upbeat or enlivened to chance; it's an intentional state that when practised regularly can become lasting levity. It enables our bodies to be placed into a feel-good state first – even if we're not feeling too flash at the time – and our mind then follows. The Laughter Effect comprises multiple elements to boost joy and create an impermeable shield of resilience to life's challenges; to prime your 'feeling' body and 'thinking' mind towards optimal mental health.

The Laughter Effect recognises that all emotions need to be experienced: the good, the not so good and even the less than not so good. That's what makes us human. It's about intentionally calling upon the energy of laughter – the essence of joy to counter stress hormones and stimulate a daily 'DOSE' of positive wellbeing: dopamine, our brain's reward centre; oxytocin, endearingly known as the molecule of love; serotonin, our body's antidepressant; and endorphins, our happy hormones. All of which you'll become more familiar with throughout this book as you get equipped with the resources that enable you to live the Laughter Effect. When applied daily, the techniques, strategies and practices you'll learn about can transform your physical, mental, social and emotional landscape. I have pieced together the philosophy that contributes to the Laughter Effect over many years, inspired by my personal and professional experience. It draws on my extensive research and practice, as well as that of other laughter and humour practitioners, together with wisdom from humour and laughter therapy, positive psychology, mindfulness and neuroscience. It is enriched by stories of personal transformation from around the globe* and some pretty serious scientific research.

LET'S GET STARTED

1. List five things that make you laugh.

2. Who are your 'go-to' people to make you laugh? In one word, how do they make you feel?

3. When is your earliest memory of laughing? Who were you with? Do you recall what you were doing? Spend a little time connecting to this joy – wrap yourself up in the sound and feel of laughter.

---

* For privacy reasons, some client names and details have been changed.

By now you may have formed an idea of the type of person you think I am. Perhaps a Pollyanna personality: naively optimistic; head in the sky. Or maybe you think I've never been touched by grief, illness or sadness? I can certainly tell you I'm not immune to these things. So, how did my exploration into the Laughter Effect begin?

About twenty years ago, I was feeling a little dejected after my proposal for a series of gluten-free, dairy-free and largely vegetarian cookbooks was rejected by numerous publishers, who deemed the 'market too small to justify the high production cost of such highly specialised cookbooks'. (Fortune tellers they were not!) I had developed a keen interest in wellbeing thanks to my history of chronic fatigue syndrome (CFS). I decided to return to study. However, to meet post-graduate university requirements, I needed some experience in the field. As luck would have it, a WHO Global Conference on Health Promotion was being hosted in Melbourne at the time; I applied and was accepted as a rapporteur contributing to the daily session wrap up. Amid the many 'serious' sessions, one stood out to me – Laughter Yoga. This I had to report on.

Seasoned facilitator Phillipa Challis outlined the fundamentals, before inviting the audience to partake in this surprisingly novel practice. As I laughed along with the other participants, I immediately felt the uplifting energy and physical and emotional transformation. It was one of the most enlivening experiences of my life. In the twenty long years I had suffered from CFS, I had consulted a multitude of medical specialists and complementary health practitioners, yet the health bounce I received from Laughter Yoga was more immediate and impactful than anything else I'd tried. I knew I had stumbled upon my destiny.

I began studying health promotion and, not long after, I trained as a Laughter Yoga leader. I became an expert extolling laughter's virtue to anyone who'd listen. That was until a distinctly un-funny time in my life – a bowel cancer diagnosis at age forty-two. Despite there being nothing humorous about cancer, I knew deep within that laughter was inextricably bound to my experience. The moment had arrived to practise what I preached. I just needed time (and a couple of major operations) to connect the dots.

The first nudge was the timing of a corporate Laughter Yoga lingerie party, where I was invited to be the facilitator. When I'd received the booking many months prior, I was tickled pink. But four days before major bowel surgery, the last place I wanted to be was surrounded by twenty or so excitable women fussing over fancy negligees. I autopiloted through the health benefits of laughter before facilitating the active laughter session. Within moments I felt lighter and brighter, and by the end, almost weightless. The endorphins (our body's internal source of morphine) kicked in and a surge of excitement for life passed through me. It was the first time I acknowledged that I had needed this remedy more than the group I was facilitating needed it. Having literally laughed much of my stress away, I was psychologically more prepared and stronger for the five-hour surgery awaiting me.

I decided I'd turn theory into practice. To turbocharge my wellbeing, I wouldn't wait until I was in the mood for laughing. In the aftermath of my surgery, I'd instigate the laughs. But little did I know! For weeks after my operation, along with 30 centimetres of my bowel, the ability to laugh was taken away from me. Delicate breaths were challenging enough. This thing I'd taken for granted my whole life had been stolen from me.

Post-op, my body felt like it had collided with a semitrailer. Feeling glum, I needed a large dose of positivity – along with another shot of morphine. As if magnetised, my hand was drawn to the pull of a nearby pencil and large white paper placemat lining my untouched breakfast tray. I began listing everything I was grateful for in my current situation, from the importance of slowing down – even if it had been enforced – to my body's miraculous capacity to heal. Overwhelmed by feelings of profound gratitude, for being alive, I was compelled to keep writing.

It wasn't long before a beaming smile lightened my face and mood. It felt like every cell, every tissue, every muscle was smiling. From darkness came light, and grief for what I'd lost was transformed into gratitude. I had totally forgotten about my pain. When the nurse came in to administer my morphine and saw me seated upright, serenely smiling, she boomeranged out of my room believing she had wandered into the wrong one. My body's natural morphine supply had kicked in. That was my 'aha' moment. I was embodying the Laughter Effect.

That's when my exploration of the Laughter Effect expanded beyond physical laughter into interrelated areas. I didn't simply want to wait to feel good, instead I sought to actively increase opportunities to intentionally intensify these feelings. I wanted to embody positivity, whether through wholehearted smiling, gratitude or priming my mind to scan for possibilities, not problems, assisted by positive journaling, where I could reframe grievances with gratitude or levity, or amplify 'micromoments' – as coined by Professor of Positive Psychology Barbara Fredrickson – of joy in my day.

. . . .

Since then, through research I've conducted into laughter therapy and by delivering countless individual and group laughter sessions for wellness programs – from aged care to corporate and government – no matter the cohort or demographic, I have marvelled at the effectiveness of the Laughter Effect and how it can be applied in a range of everyday scenarios: traffic jams, a spat with your partner, and even a pandemic. Developing neural pathways towards meeting life's stresses with more levity takes practice and time, like any muscle-building exercise. The Laughter Effect gives your body and mind a workout. How much of a workout is entirely up to you.

I've written this book with the goal to inspire change in your life and encourage daily practice to promote positive wellbeing. To awaken your inner and outer smile; unleash the power of your sixth sense, humour;

and authentically amplify and build positive emotions. This book aims to provide a laughter lens with which to view the world and add a new dimension to a range of self-care and wellbeing strategies, including mindfulness, gratitude and self-compassion, empowering people who practise it to lead healthier and happier lives.

We'll dive into the history of laughter, assess its evolutionary role in human survival – or as I prefer to think of it, 'thrival' (survival + thrive) – and create a framework for achieving the positive things you want in life. And we'll address the question: *Is laughter really the best medicine?* By the end, you'll be equipped with fundamental life and laugh skills through an exploration of intentional laughter practices. The two main modalities we'll look at are Laughter Yoga and Laughter Wellness – laughing for the health, and not simply for the humour, of it – and we'll also delve into the neuroscience of smiling, embrace gratitude to create a shift in life perspective, and explore how being kinder and more self-compassionate is a vital inner resource.

Throughout the book you'll find smiling and laughter activities, mindfulness practices and positive journaling techniques to create a 'laughter mindset'. You'll be introduced to your friendly Serotonin Sister – an upbeat incarnation of Dear Abby – who'll provide uplifting and enlightening solutions to commonly posed dilemmas. There's room for reflection and opportunities to connect to your playful side. Before you turn each page or move onto a new chapter, please consider building in some mindful pauses. This will help to enrich your read and enable any positive emotion or feel-good sensations to wash over you.

There are practical tips in the back of the book – The Laughter Effect in Practice – that will help you connect to your laughter-side in all areas of your life.

This book is about investing in yourself so that no matter what comes your way, resourced with the tools of the Laughter Effect, you'll be able to respond with greater equanimity. Over time, you'll notice you're laughing and smiling more – saying yes to wholehearted living. Your resilience to stress will be enhanced, enabling you to bounce forward from adversity with humour, levity and grace.

Finally, if you feel the need for permission to activate your own Laughter Effect, consider it granted. It's time to cultivate the brighter side of life – to awaken your inner sparkle and shine.

In love and laughter,
Ros

1

The History of Laughter

God has a smile on His face
—Psalm 42:5

Laughter, humour and joy are vital in life, and have guided us mere mortals through plagues, climate change–induced floods, and the destruction caused by the untamed egos of dictators. So, let's begin by dispelling any myths regarding humour and laughter's therapeutic value as hippy, trippy or New Age. That is, unless you believe Adam and Eve to be so. The genesis of the Laughter Effect in Judaeo-Christian traditions is, conveniently, in the Old Testament's Genesis.

The Bible is called the 'Good Book' with reason. Amid the many fire and brimstone moments in it are multiple references to happiness as the real source of wealth. The Old Testament is a veritable repository of meme-able gems hinting at laughter's therapeutic value. 'A merry heart doeth good like a medicine: but a broken spirit drieth the bones.' (Proverbs 17:22) 'Then was our mouth filled with laughter' (Psalms 126:2), a mirthful expression of redemption and joy and gratitude to God. 'Blessed are you who weep now, for you shall laugh!' (Luke 6:21) Such statements could easily be assumed to be attributed to meditation guru Deepak Chopra or the Dalai Lama, but are as old as time itself.

Stories that reflect the application of the Laughter Effect infuse the Bible, including matriarch Sarah, childless until aged ninety, who on discovering her pregnancy pronounced, 'God has brought me laughter, and everyone who hears about this will laugh with me.' (Genesis 21:6) The son she bears, on instruction from God, is given the name Yitzhak (Isaac), meaning 'to laugh' in Hebrew. Isaac's life was far from a laugh, traversing the precipice of misfortune, although he survived adversity with unexpected joy.

Turning to the Muslim world and Islam, there are accounts of Mohammed laughing and making others laugh. Anas b. Mālik, the Prophet's servant until his death, informed that: 'The Prophet was one of the men who joked the most.'[1] He was constantly seen smiling, and taught that smiling in the face of one another's brother is charity. Moderation, laughter and lightheartedness were also advocated in the Sunnahs – a model based on the Prophet's teachings and practices – to lighten burdens, bring joy to oneself and others, and ease anxiety.

The Laughter Effect wasn't only crucial to Judaeo-Christian-Islamic traditions; it was also an important attribute of many ancient civilisations and indigenous cultures. So intrinsic was humour and laughter to Aboriginal and Torres Strait Islander peoples, it is embedded in their Dreaming stories of creation, dating back at least 65,000 years. The Kamilaroi people of northern New South Wales and southern Queensland say Venus occasionally twinkles when it's low in the sky. They believe it's an old man who told a rude joke and has been laughing ever since. Twentieth-century First Nations activist and poet Oodgeroo Noonuccal , also known as Kath Walker, articulated the Indigenous laughing connection to Country as: 'We are the wonder tales of Dream Time, the tribal legends told ... We are the past, the hunts and the laughing games ...'

Many activities encouraged laughter in Indigenous Australian cultures, from swimming games to football. There was also playful communication, talking 'gibberish', tickling, giggling and laughing play.

Ceremonial clowns helped settle old feuds and maintain social control, often painting themselves as animals and infusing poignant messages in dance and entertainment. A man noted for his clownish abilities would assume a primary role in bringing peace to quarrelling parties, pretending to spear the offenders, spurring a hilarious response from the rest of the tribe. The ensuing loud laughter prevented the angry parties from committing overt acts of rage or causing further trouble.[2] There were very few ritual occasions where laughter and joking were out of place. Sadly, since colonisation, traditional Indigenous games have been largely lost.

Laughter was integral to many indigenous people's social fabric all over the world. Mythical 'tricksters' featured in the stories of nearly every Native American tribe. These tricksters would tell stories dictating acceptable and unacceptable tribal behaviour, and while they may have been practical jokers, they were believed to possess supernatural powers. Tricksters assumed a spiritual role in ceremonial practice, harnessing the upheld belief of humour's ability to implement change and to heal.[3] They commandeered the Laughter Effect, often botching their tricks, to ramp up laughter.

In addition to tricksters, almost every tribe had a personal clown or two. Working alongside a medicine man, clowns ranked third on a tribe's totem pole. The Hunkpapa Sioux had both 'happiness' clowns and 'sadness' clowns, who contributed to the emotional wellbeing of individual tribal members by performing dances within sacred ceremonies. The 'sadness' clown helped diminish feelings of depression, while the 'happiness' clown enhanced joy. It was believed that dual clowns upheld a community's spiritual balance. They were afforded a freedom to express emotions that many other members of the community could not. Social critics of the highest order, their mimicry and joking exposed hypocrisy and arrogance, quelling inappropriate behaviour and helping to maintain a healthy social dynamic.

According to a Native American elder known as 'Granny':

In the days before the invaders came … we had clowns. Not clowns like you see now, with round red noses and baggy costumes. Our clowns wore all kinds of stuff. Anythin' they felt like, they wore. And they didn't just come out once in a while to act silly and make people laugh, our clowns were with us all the time, as important to the village as the chief, or the shaman, or the dancers, or the poets.[4]

As in First Nations culture in Australia, across the Arctic laughter was the ultimate icebreaker in many Canadian Inuit games, too. They played laughing games to brighten spirits during the long, bleak winter months. One favourite was Animal muk, where participants form a circle with one person standing in the middle who uses only animal sounds or actions to make someone in the outside circle smile or laugh. If the person in the circle smiles, laughs or breaks eye contact, they will take their turn in the middle to try to make someone else in the circle smile or laugh.[5] In most games, a desire to find pleasure in the game was just as important as winning.

Laughter was intentionally encouraged and initiated, demonstrating a person's ability to control emotions and maintain composure. Laughter is also a prime feature of Inuit throat singing, *katajjaq*, where two women face one another at close quarters, with no instrumental accompaniment, and sing a duet. Bursts of laughter mingle with bursts of song – a natural expression of feel-good vibes, and an appreciation of a partner's performance. The practice is experiencing a resurgence after being quashed for many years by Christian missionaries. Inuit culture considered laughter to be *igloo* (i-glue) of society. An old Inuit adage affirms: 'Those who know how to play can easily leap over the adversities of life. And one who can sing and laugh never brews mischief.'[6]

LAUGHTER TRADITIONS

Do you have any laughter traditions that have been passed down through the generations?

At each annual family Jewish Passover Seder ritual, one of the final songs of the evening is 'Chad Gadya' ('One Little Goat'). No matter the hour, it's a sure-fire way to generate peals of laughter, as everyone is randomly assigned a sound effect. The repetition in each stanza underscores the ebb and flow of Jewish history as told by an array of characters – cat, goat, dog, stick, fire, water, ox, Angel of Death and the Holy One, Blessed be He. The song reminds me of one particular Seder at a friend's house. The cat sound effect was so realistic (I take full credit!) that their tiny yelping dog hurtled onto the table to chase the 'cat'. You can probably imagine what the table looked like afterwards – it was 'cat'astrophic!

We now move from igloos to pyramids, where in Ancient Egypt, pharaohs and queens were entertained by jesters and buffoons. It's also considered the home of the world's oldest joke.[7] A fart joke – I kid you not – from the Sumerian civilisation in 1900BC, captured in perpetuity on papyrus: 'Something which has never occurred since time immemorial; a young woman did not fart in her husband's lap.'

And here's a joke I'd like to contribute:

How did Cleopatra feel when she learnt she was queen of Egypt?
She was in denial (de-Nile, get it?).

Ancient Eastern civilisations also employed the Laughter Effect. Across China, Korea and Japan there were dedicated words for jesters, acrobats, jugglers and entertainers. In China, records of laughter rituals date back to the Shang dynasty (1600–1050 BC). *Huaji*, a portmanteau of *hua* (slippery) and *ji* (a bobbling motion), were performers who wore asymmetrical red-and-black costumes and delighted in an assortment of frenzied activities to uplift and entertain. Their efforts were deemed indispensable, mediating between emperors on earth and the heavens above, hoping to establish good relations for the recently deceased.

In Korea, trickster tigers are considered an important figure in folklore and were common at festivals, wreaking havoc with backfiring tricks, resulting in laughter. And if you thought drinking games were a new addition to the party scene, think again. Korea heralds the world's oldest drinking game, *juryeonggu*. An archaeological dig in the 1970s uncovered a fourteen-sided dice dating to around the seventh century CE. Side 4's instructions translate as, *Drink a big cup and laugh loudly*, taking the notion of keeping ancestral spirits happy to a whole new level.

We now turn to a country that has gifted us karaoke, Nintendo, anime and sushi, among many other things – Japan. In the *Warai Matsuri* – a festival celebrated to this day in the town of Hidakagawa in the Wakayama prefecture – a clown called *Suzu-furi* holds a bell and makes people laugh, together with shouting, 'Laughing! Laughing!' Laughing is believed to push evil spirits away.

From the ancient East to Ancient Greece, where epic poet Homer, not of *The Simpsons*, wrote 2800 years ago in passages in the *Iliad* and the *Odyssey* that Mount Olympus was said to ring with the laughter of the gods as 'the exuberance of their celestial joy after their daily banquet'. In the *Odyssey*, Odysseus tells the Cyclops that his real name is 'Nobody'. When Odysseus instructs his men to attack the Cyclops, the Cyclops shouts, 'Help, nobody is attacking me!' No one came to help. It's like a line from Abbott and Costello's rapid-fire 'Who's on First' sketch.

As part of the healing process, Greek physicians used to prescribe a visit to the hall of comedians. Can you imagine if physicians suggested that today? The Ancient Greeks can even boast their very own 'Laughing Philosopher', Democritus – known for laughing at human follies. In addition to being one of the founders of ancient atomist theory, he sought to understand what makes one happy, declaring happiness and cheerfulness to be the highest, noblest goal of everyone. It would be hard to find a more cheerful and twinkly eyed individual than Democritus. Curious? Google his image. However, his cheery disposition raised a few eyebrows in his hometown, Abdera. So much so that residents called upon the great doctor Hippocrates – of the famed Hippocratic oath – to assess whether Democritus's frequent laughter was pathological and a form of madness. Surely such a state was unnatural?

Next up is Ancient Rome, where we come to lawyer, statesman and writer Cicero, well known for his wit. Roman judgement decreed he was 'far too funny for his own good'. Indeed, Cicero was classified as 'a laughter addict'. He believed humour to be a defining feature of sociability that enhanced relationships, enforced shared community norms and strengthened one's public figure. You might be wondering, *What have the Romans ever done for us?* Well, aside from aqueducts, irrigation, sewerage, education, roads, medicine and wine, they also gave us the world's first-documented joke book – the *Philogelos* (or *Laughter Lover*), a compendium of gags dating to the fourth or fifth century CE. Some still have legs and are rehashed by comedians today. One refers to a famous retort spouted by Herod Archelaus. The Court barber, a known chatterbox, asked him, 'How should I cut your hair?' Archelaus responded: 'In silence.'

Several hundred years later, the Roman emperor was gone, but laughter remained – a challenge for the Roman Catholic Church, which did its darndest to extinguish joy. Paradoxically, it was medieval monks who were tasked with transcribing the 260 or so jokes from the *Philogelos*.

The Romans demonstrated a penchant for gallows humour, guffawing over contemporary issues of the day, such as crucifixion. Another laughter legend hailing from Roman times is April Fools' Day, tracing back to the ancient holiday of Hilaria. This confirms a suspicion of mine that if there were a Humour God, he/she/they would most definitely be called Hilarios. It seems the Romans always looked on the bright side of life.

In the thirteenth century, inspired by Aristotle, Saint Thomas Aquinas decreed laughter permissible for Christians under certain spiritual conditions. It was sanctioned owing to it being a distinctly human behaviour, and not as bestial and animalistic as many critics believed. Little did they know, centuries later there would be a revolutionary discovery about all manner of creatures displaying laughter, including rats.

Even the royals were fond of a laugh. Richard Tarleton, a court jester, was said to have kept Queen Elizabeth I in better health than her physicians. When she was out of good humour, he would lighten her mood, curing her melancholy better than all of her physicians.[8] And another queen, Mary, was introduced to laughter as a cure early in life. Plagued with ill health, Mary received a letter from her mother, Katherine of Aragon, which revealed, 'a little comfort and mirth should undoubtedly be half a health unto her. I have proved the like by experience being diseased of the same infirmary and know how much good it may do.'[9] Jane Fool, Queen Mary I's entrusted companion for at least twenty years, was so invaluable to her mistresses' wellbeing that she was gifted a wardrobe smarter than the Queen's own courtesans.

Without the scientific knowledge we have now, jesters unwittingly dispensed a DOSE of dopamine, oxytocin, serotonin and endorphins. It was a jovial time for jesters, who were often afforded lead roles in Shakespeare's plays. The most famous was *King Lear*'s fool, who functions as the king's inner conscience. In the play, the fool is described as 'a fellow of infinite jest, of most excellent fancy'. Often wise and intelligent, Shakespeare's fools were believed to be The Bard's mouthpiece, shining a light on pertinent issues. *A Hundred Merry Tales*, also known as *Shakespeare's Jestbook*, was first printed in 1526 and is the earliest known example of an English jestbook. Bulging with uncouth yet witty tales of foolhardy and hypocritical clergymen, vulgar women and dim Welshman, it was even reputed to have been read to Queen Elizabeth I on her deathbed. One can but hope she passed with a smile on her face.

Prior to Britain's industrial revolution, Cornish chemist Humphry Davy and his boss, English physician Thomas Beddoes, gathered in a drawing room. They were ruminating over which gases might be important for lung health. The specific gas in question was nitrous oxide. Far from sterile, Davy's laboratory was the place to be. Poets, playwrights, doctors and scientists congregated at his famed N_2O (nitrous oxide) parties. Yes, you read correctly. Guests were offered a puff of nitrous oxide – also known as laughing gas – from a green silk bag. These scientific experiments formed part of the early research into how nitrous oxide impacted the brain, leading to one of the most significant medical advances of the nineteenth century: anaesthesia. Guests described states of ecstasy and involuntary laughter, shouting: "Give me more, give me more; this is the most pleasurable thing I've ever experienced." Whilst [others] were running up and down the stairs and all around the house, saying odd things that they'd forget later."[10]

In those instances the effect was induced, but you'll be relieved to know that in the coming chapters I'll be sharing with you tools that will enable you to naturally access the benefits of laughter, without the need for you to get sky high on N_2O.

During the nineteenth century, English naturalist Charles Darwin devoted substantial time to researching the effects of laughter, so much so that it's surprising he's not better known for the evolutionary aspect of smiling and laughter. Darwin wanted to create a visual depiction of laughter in action. However, photographic point-and-snap moments were still decades away, and the lengthy exposure time required to capture movement would have resulted in blurry photographs. Instead, he leaned on contemporaries of the time, including French neurologist Guillaume Duchenne, who had collated an extensive photographic collection of people smiling. (More on his rather appalling methods later.) Duchenne kept a pet monkey and told his buddy Darwin that he'd often seen it smile. In an informal borrow-a-pet-monkey scheme, Darwin conducted his own empirical experiments, and delighted in noting their laughter as well as their smiles.

If a young chimpanzee be tickled – and the armpits are particularly sensitive to tickling, as in the case of our children – a more decided

chuckling or laughing sound is uttered; though the laughter is sometimes noiseless. The corners of the mouth are then drawn backwards;
and this sometimes causes the lower eyelids to be slightly wrinkled ...
The teeth in the upper jaw in the chimpanzee are not exposed when
they utter their laughing noise, in which respect they differ from us.
But their eyes sparkle and grow brighter.

Darwin's discoveries set him apart from Aristotle, who had claimed
humans were the only creatures who laughed. Fascinated with human
laughter, Darwin meticulously noted laughter's visceral effect on body
and mind:

During excessive laughter the whole body is often thrown back-
ward and shakes, or is almost convulsed. The respiration is much
disturbed; the head and face become gorged with blood, with the
veins distended; and the orbicular muscles are spasmodically con-
tracted in order to protect the eyes. Tears are freely shed ... hence ...
it is scarcely possible to point out any difference between the tear-
stained face of a person after a paroxysm of excessive laughter and
after a bitter crying-fit.[11]

Documenting what we now know as the Laughter Effect, Darwin
hung out with chimpanzees, observing that during moderate laughter there was hardly any contraction of the muscles around the eyes.
He also noticed apes didn't shed any tears when they laughed, concluding
tears of laughter to be a definitive human feature. He observed blind and
deaf individuals engaging in laughter without ever having heard or seen it,
proving it to be an innate behaviour. Darwin also noted that an expression
of intense joy leads to various purposeless movements – to dancing about,
clapping the hands, stamping, and to loud laughter. No wonder so many
institutions tried to keep a lid on laughter. Dancing can lead not only to
sex but – shock! horror! – to laughter too.

His combined body of work suggests laughter is inherently linked to our evolution from primates to higher-order species. So, as the latest in this chain of evolution, let's get laughing – there's a genetic imperative.

· · · · · · · ·

In the 1930s and 1940s, during the worst of the polio epidemic, certain US hospitals hired magicians, circus clowns and singers to entertain children who were strapped to iron lungs for over two weeks. While their bodies were immobilised, their lungs and facial muscles got a laughter workout. A mini uplift from their bleak reality.

What does a gelotologist do?

a. Develops specialty Italian ice cream

b. Constructs wobbly desserts

c. Studies humour and laughter

It is, as I'm sure most of you would have guessed, c. studies humour and laughter. Gelotology comes from the Greek root *gelos*, meaning 'to laugh'.

Grooving along to the Swinging '60s, we see the formal establishment of the science of laughter in March 1964 by sociolinguist Dr Edith Trager – naming it Gelotology. From here, Dr William Fry, professor of Psychology at Stanford University, California, took the laughter baton. Known as the Father of Gelotology, Fry published several landmark studies on the physiology of laughter in the 1970s. One equated laughter to 'internal jogging', finding that one minute of laughter was equivalent to ten minutes on the rowing machine. So, if you want to get fit, get laughing, which we'll be discussing further in chapter three.

Someone not getting their equivalent of ten minutes of laughter, or doing much swinging, was Dr Norman Cousins. In 1964, he lay in a hospital immobilised from the debilitating illness ankylosing spondylitis, a form of arthritis affecting the spine. At his worst, Cousins was nearly incapable of moving his jaw. Refusing to accept his doctor's death sentence, he took his healing into his own hands. Drawing inspiration from books describing how negative emotions, such as frustration and suppressed rage, were linked to adrenal exhaustion, Cousins assumed the opposite to be true – that positive emotions such as love, hope and faith would generate health benefits. He'd also studied brain chemistry and had more than a hunch that laughter therapy could help.

With the blessing of his treating practitioner, Cousins discharged himself from hospital, hired a nurse and checked into a hotel. Supplementing mega quantities of vitamin C with doses of comedy – E.B. White's *A Subtreasury of American Humor*, *Candid Camera*, the Marx Brothers, and Laurel and Hardy – he later wrote: 'I made the joyous discovery that ten minutes of genuine belly laughter had an anaesthetic effect and would give me at least two hours of pain-free sleep.' To the astonishment of his treating physician and the medical establishment, Cousins made a miraculous recovery and spent the next twenty years or so teaching the merits of humour and laughter in healing at the University College of Los Angeles (UCLA). Working with cancer patients, Cousins' studies found that a patient's sense of wellbeing could positively affect the functioning of the immune system and the production of cancer-fighting T-cells. His groundbreaking book, *Anatomy of an Illness* (1979), based on his own experiences, set the scene for today's burgeoning research into humour and laughter.

In 2021, Hunter Doherty 'Patch' Adams, the world's most famous clown doctor, was nominated for a Nobel Peace Prize. He has gone where no other doctor has gone. His playful antics inspired the 1998 movie *Patch Adams* starring the late legendary comedian, Robin Williams. The film is based on Patch's own challenges with mental illness and his health journey, which led him to conclude that 'the patient is the doctor too'. His outlandish methods, taking the clown out of the circus and into a hospital ward, clashed with the medical establishment, and in 1971 he took laughter matters into his own hands and established the Gesundheit! Institute in West Virginia. He transformed thousands of lives by dispensing love and laughter to promote healing and wellbeing. He was a visionary, and in 1984 when funding gave up, he didn't.

Dressed in colourful clothing, full of compassion and equipped with bubbles galore, Patch gathered a team of Gesundheit Global Outreach Clowns (GO!CLOWNS), and beginning in the former Soviet Union in 1985, used 'red nasal diplomacy' to transport the Laughter Effect into hospitals, orphanages, aged care institutions and onto the streets. With his merry band of medical clowns, he developed clinics to provide humanitarian and medical care in the most distressed regions, and performed in over seventy countries. Wonderful for around 90 per cent of the general population. Not so great for the remaining minority who suffered from coulrophobia.

What is coulrophobia?

a. Intense dislike of cauliflower

b. Fear of clowns

c. Fear of being confined in an enclosed space

If you guessed b, you're right: fear of clowns.

Coulrophobia stems from the ancient Greek word, *coulro*, for 'one who goes on stilts'. Symptoms of coulrophobia include sweating, nausea, feelings of dread, fast heartbeat, crying, screaming, or anger at being placed in a situation where a clown is present.

From oversized shoes and doses of slapstick, we now subtract the comedic side of laughter therapy to reveal the newest kid on the block,

Laughter Yoga. This primary contemporary non-humour-based laughter practice challenges the assumption that a smile or laugh needs to be externally generated, or relies on a humorous situation to generate laughter. Instead, it focuses on laughing for the health of it, where the laughter begins first in the body, which then influences the mind, and in doing so, changes its biochemistry. As we will explore further, this has a positive influence on body, mind and soul.

Popularised in India by Dr Madan Kataria (also known as Dr K) in 1995, Laughter Yoga is steeped in Eastern philosophy. It combines pranayama deep breathing exercises, clapping, chanting *ho ho, ha ha ha*, and simulated laughter exercises. You don't have to travel to India to laugh it up, Laughter Yoga has become a burgeoning worldwide movement with over tens of thousands of dedicated physical clubs and online sessions. It's an ideal antidote to our stress-filled lives, or when laughter is the last thing in the world we feel like doing, such as during illness or other challenging personal circumstances.

. . . .

From biblical times to the present, from cultures steeped in mysticism to Western civilisations, laughter's ripple effect is far and wide. That's not to say there haven't been killjoys along the way, however the innate gift of laughter wins, keeping individuals and cultures strong and resilient. The world would be a different place had it not been for the Laughter Effect. As the psalmists write – 'He who sits in heaven shall laugh.' Or as I'd posit, laughter is the ultimate expression of heaven on earth.

2

We Laugh to ~~Survive~~ Thrive

He who laughs, lasts

—Mary Pettibone Poole

The Laughter Effect, encompassing the humble smile, can be witnessed in the earliest stages of our development. We *ha ha* before we *da da* or *ma ma*. No matter what your background, age or where you're situated in the world, we all smile and laugh in the same language. A smile or shared laugh satiates an evolutionary survival role. It's a critical inner resource bestowed to every one of us. A visual demonstration of love, a smile optimises our chances of survival by enhancing bonding with our caregivers and increasing the chance of timely attention. It's, therefore, no surprise that laughter and humour were fundamental to human evolution.

The more positive early smiling and laughter interactions with main caregivers are, the safer and more loved a child feels. It lays the foundation for managing emotional responses through life. The stronger this laughter/smiling 'scaffolding' is, the better, otherwise a few bad experiences may result in it tumbling down, like a Jenga tower. This can lead to feeling less confident to laugh freely without fear of judgement, and create an unconscious suppression of laughter. Households dominated by anger, disinterest or disengagement often have fewer opportunities for a child to 'muck around', play and laugh. The Laughter Effect contributes to a calmer and more loving atmosphere in a household, which increases the chances of functional relationships later in life.[1]

I am indebted with gratitude for the significant role laughter has played in my life, both in my earlier emotional attachment to others and attachment to my own children. This is something I realised more than ever when my second son came into the world with sound lungs, cavernous enough to play the trumpet (which he later did). My first night alone with him in the hospital, I was gazing adoringly at this little miracle, wondering what he should be named. I was still astounded by his entry into the world, amniotic sac intact, when he smiled (which may or may not have been caused by wind) and it was decided. Like his biblical ancestor, and great-grandfathers on both sides, this boy would assume the name Zak, short for Yitzchak – meaning 'to laugh'. It was a visionary choice: without seeing that smile of his, I would have cracked under the pressure of eight tortuous croupy months.

Anytime he shared a gummy smile, or tiny chuckle – ZAP! – the sleepless nights, endless stream of nappies and indiscriminate crying were forgotten, and I was back under love's spell, at his beck and call. That's what happens – clever little beings. My dopamine, oxytocin, serotonin and endorphins went wild thanks to Zak's wide smile.

Behaviourally, first comes smiling, then comes a baby's first laugh – a reassuring and joyful sign that bub is healthy, happy and all is well. It's a joyful feedback loop enhancing connection and affection, a moment captured for posterity in a baby journal (or by today's parenting generation, on Twitter, Instagram or TikTok – or all the above). However, nothing compares to the Native American Navajo's (known as the Diné) First Laugh Ceremony, *A'wee Chi'deedloh*. To the Navajo, a baby's first laugh is seen as a sign of the baby transcending their spiritual existence and indicating readiness to join their family and community in life and love. From around three months of age, caregivers and other family members compete with one another to elicit the first hallowed laugh by tickling, peek-a-booing, poking and silly faces. Whoever wins hosts a First Laugh Ceremony to celebrate the successful transition of the baby into the world. As a mark of respect to the family they're born into and to honour the spiritual world, the baby is considered the ceremonial host, and each guest receives a plate of food, rock salt (symbolising tears shed through loss or sadness and connection to the earth) and a bag of goodies. The expressed desire is that the baby will always experience togetherness among family and friends throughout life.

Laughter is a social beast – always greedy for company. In a study of preschool children, on average they laughed at cartoons eight times more when in the company of others compared to when they were alone, and smiled almost three times as much.[2] Laughter's social bonding role enhances connection between adults and children, and encourages them to be fully present in each other's company. That is, unless the caregiver is distracted, not by their infant's animated face but by an inanimate screen. It doesn't take long for a child to assess their lack of engagement as disinterest. One study found an infant's expression switches to 'time out' if their emotional state is unacknowledged for more than three seconds.[3] A mere three seconds! But from an infant's perspective, that's a lifetime. Our attention is constantly hijacked by text messages, email pings, Snapchat; the list goes on. Where does this leave our young'uns? Can we multitask parenting in the digital era? For a baby or young infant's social development, eye contact and one's full attention is crucial. Yet, increasingly, playgrounds are filled with children on play equipment while nearby parents or caregivers are wrapped up in their phones. We can't always give 100 per cent of our attention to our kids all the time, but we need to be wary that in the count of *one cat and dog, two cat and dog, three cat and dog*, a precious moment of connection may be lost.

Developing our laugh-print

Children learn by modelling other's behaviour, and the style of laughter they pick up is one such behaviour. Not only do we have our unique voice and speaking style, but we also have our very own 'laugh-print'. It's as individual as we are, and shaped by our environment. A louder style of laughter might be a requisite to capture attention in a raucous household, while in a less bustling home, laughter could be whispered yet still achieve the desired attention. Over the years, people have shared with me their familial laugh-prints. One of the most humorous was a woman who married into a family where the three brothers and father all shared the same laugh – that of the mangy cartoon dog Precious Pupp, from where the famous wheezy Muttley laugh derives. And another woman told me that, to her amazement, her daughter had a replica guffaw of her grandfather's, whom her daughter had only met a handful of times.

Across cultures we guffaw, chuckle, chortle, howl, snigger, roar, snort, titter, hoot, whoop, snicker and cackle – the latter assumedly deriving from the word cachinnate (cack-innate), which means to laugh loudly. (Where has that gem of a word been hiding my whole life?) Our cultural background shapes our laugh-print. Many Asian cultures have an introverted laugh-print. Social etiquette dictates, especially for women, that it's far more polite to titter behind one's hands, as bearing one's teeth is 'unlady-like'. A common practice in several Asian countries was for women to dye their teeth black (known in Japanese as *ohaguro*), regarded as both a status symbol and a way of preventing tooth decay. While this practice has largely gone out of vogue, perhaps in part it has served to evolutionarily decommission a toothy grin? Confucianism, which teaches that public displays of emotion should be repressed to 'save face', has influenced Korean etiquette. Not only do many Korean women cover their mouths whenever they laugh or smile, but to this day many turn their heads away from others.

This is in stark contrast to the Mbuti people of the Ituri Forest, located in the Democratic Republic of the Congo. Their laugh-print is physical to the extreme. British-American anthropologist and writer Colin Turnbull, the only Western writer known to have witnessed the Mbuti laughing, observed them lying down and kicking their legs in the air, panting and shaking in outbursts of hilarity. While this might seem exuberant, for these indigenous people it is their norm.

Over a lifetime we're exposed to a litany of laughs, but we all have our go-to laugh. I'm a giggler and have been ever since my Giggling Gertie school days. There are scenario-based laughs – embarrassed, silent, flirtatious, piercing, relief, anxious, acoustic, to name just a few. Then there's the snorter, the person who laughs so hard they snort, and then laugh because they snorted. That behaviour has a name: snaughling. I love snaughlers!

Involuntary laughter

As laughter is a behaviour not under conscious control, for the most part, we might conclude that it can't be that complex and it's taken for granted.

Yet laughter is one of the most complicated things our bodies process, making laughing as an infant, before the brain has fully developed, and at life's closing curtain, when, for many, cognitive functions have diminished, even more remarkable. It's a largely involuntary neurological process: our brain decides, based on what it sees or hears, whether it's in a laughing mood. It doesn't bother consulting with manual thought processes, which can be a tad embarrassing if you're at a work lunch and someone says something a little inappropriate or uproarious during the meal. Before your sensibilities kick in, laughter erupts from your mouth and even your nostrils. Blame your hippocampus, not your colleague. Part of five areas of the human brain involved in the production of laughter and assessment of humour, the hippocampus is one of the key players that determines our emotional responses. Another top dog is the frontal lobe of the brain and the limbic system, consisting of the hippocampus, amygdala, thalamus and hypothalamus. The frontal lobe is divided into left and right hemispheres. Lefty determines which sounds, images or experiences are funny. Our creative Righty determines if a situation or joke is funny or not.

The limbic system is a legacy of our ancient primal brain, responsible for basic emotions such as fear, anger and pleasure. It's involved in the body's responses necessary for human survival, including feeding, fighting, fleeing and an expletive also beginning with 'f' associated with reproduction. It takes its cue from the frontal lobe, assessing whether 'to laugh, or not to laugh', as Shakespeare may've put it. Either signalling the physical process of laughter into motion, or not. The more we laugh, the more powerful a workout our limbic system receives.

Taking laughing matters into your own hands

As we enter the Age of Maturity – aka adulthood – the more we need to take laughing matters into our own hands. If you google, *How many times children laugh in a day versus adults*, some results will proclaim anything from 300–400 times, whereas adults is only ten to twelve. I'm yet to find evidence to support this claim. In the few studies I have found that examined laughter frequency in both children and adults, the laughs do not add up.

In my pursuit to find out average daily laughter, a question I pose to many of my audiences is: *How many times on average do you laugh in a day?* I'm asking about laugh-out-loud moments, as opposed to a solitary *ha* or laughing on the inside (LOTI). I find that most audience members rarely, if ever, consider how frequently they laugh.

MEASURE YOUR LAUGHTER FREQUENCY

How many times on average do you laugh in a day?

Is there a difference between weekdays and weekends?

What conditions enable you to have a bumper laughter day?

I have found two demographics consistently reach and excel the ten to twelve times per day: early childhood educators and lifestyle staff in residential aged care. Merriment is integral to their day jobs. Especially children's environments, which are generally highly conducive to laughter, with plentiful eye contact and close proximity by sitting knee-to-knee on a classroom floor or at shared or closely aligned desks.

So why is it that children in general laugh so much more than adults? Hundreds of reasons have been expounded to me over the years: children don't have mortgages or responsibilities or a lot of stress; children are less self-conscious, see things for the first time, live in the moment, are uninhibited; adults have to work, or they take themselves too seriously.

There's truth in most of these assessments, but it's a misnomer that children's lives are devoid of stress. They may not have adult stress, but they have 'kid stress': someone snatching their lunch; a bully teasing them; perhaps a parent or caregiver is rarely home, so they miss out on vital bonding, reading, play or bath time; or they live in an environment characterised by bickering and not enough love. Stress accompanies every stage of life.

What has yet to develop in childhood is the layer of critical analysis adults apply to laughing. With conditioning also rises a sense of vulnerability: that feeling of being naked and exposed when we let loose or are silly. In response, we modify our thoughts and actions for fear of what people may think about us, rather than acting as we would if no one were watching or judging.

Children laugh from the heart. They don't think about it, they just do it. In adults, laughter becomes an intellectual construct from the head.

While laughter is a subconscious, innate behaviour, over time and in response to cues from our external environment regarding social mores, our conscious mind overrides the free-spirited nature of laughter. We *think* laughter and don't *do* laughter. We weigh up the benefit or deficit of laughing out of turn. *Is it appropriate to laugh now? What will people think of me? I'm sure they're laughing at me, not with me. I'm in a serious job now and my boss will think less of me if it seems I'm having too much fun.* And so it goes until, over time, our laugh-out-loud response becomes more and more subdued and repressed. Then one day, we're exposed to a humorous scenario, and guess what? Do we laugh? Nope. We have gone so far down the rabbit hole of seriosity that instead of an outburst of laughter, out spurts, 'That's funny!' Or if something even funnier happens, this clincher, 'That's really funny!' It's not just our lunch that's been stolen: it's the uninhibited ability to express our natural state of joy.

. . . .

In the hundreds of laughter programs I've delivered over the years, I've asked participants not only how many times a day on average they laugh, but also why they like to laugh and how laughter makes them feel. Whether they were government employees, bank managers, teachers, cleaners, children, older people, sick or healthy, several common themes emerged. A wide range of reasons were given, including that it makes people feel good; that it's fun, relaxing and stress relieving; it results in feeling alive and energised; it puts them in a good mood; laughing reminds them of childhood and distracts from the worries of the world; it helps them forget problems; it helps them to focus, sleep, connect with others better; and sometimes because it's better than the alternative – crying. In one session, one participant even described a good laugh as a 'mind orgasm'!

Yet one response stood out by a scientific mile: 'Because it makes me happy.'

SEROTONIN SISTER

I recall a time in my life when I was laughed at, which made me feel really uncomfortable. What's the best strategy to draw on if once again I feel this happening?

Most people have experienced this at some point during their lives. Try not to focus on the negative laughter experience. Remind yourself it was one moment in time. Instead, ease back to your laughter-side (the aspect of yourself that laughs freely and is aligned to levity) by expressing it when you're in non-judgemental, loving company. Perhaps you can even get to a point where you can find the funny (or absurdity) in being laughed at?

This is where it gets interesting. If laughter is a shortcut to happiness, why don't we do more of it? We want to be happy – we crave it. 'Life, Liberty and the pursuit of Happiness' is even written into the United States Declaration of Independence. Why, then, is laughter left to chance or forgotten? Is it like a diet that we know is good for us, do for a while, then give up on? Or perhaps it's because there are fewer opportunities for social engagement in our increasingly 'me-centric' as opposed to 'we-centric' society. We're more socially isolated. We live in an era where smartphones, laptops and tablets replace cinemas or familial lounge-room TV viewing. In cubicled workplaces, faces are hidden behind a screen/computer monitor with minimal social interaction, and in recent times, more people are working from home (WFH), virtually engaging with work colleagues, with water-cooler opportunities for incidental laughter diminished. The other tablet we are increasingly reaching for is the round white pharmaceutical variety – a means to numb our pain and restore equilibrium.

. . . .

Life isn't always a barrel of laughs. It wasn't designed to be. If we were laughing all the time, as exhilarating as that may sound, not only would it be exhausting, but there would also be no demarcation between life's highs and lows. Eventually you'd need to top LOL experiences with more laughter, to make them stand out. This can be explained by what professor of psychology Sonja Lyubomirsky refers to as our 'happiness set point'. If something good happens your sense of happiness rises, and if something bad happens it falls, but after a while it normalises back to whatever your set point is.[4]

Or as I prefer to reframe as 'The Zebra Equation'. As a child, I tagged along to one of my dad's medical conferences in South Africa. We went on a safari – a once-in-a-lifetime experience. There were hoots of delight when we saw our first zebra – click, click, click went our cameras. Yet after a while, no matter how many zebras were in view, it was, meh,

SEROTONIN SISTER

I used to laugh lots but now I rarely do. How can I connect more to my laughter-side?

This is one of the most common questions I'm asked. The accumulation of stress impacts our daily laughter quotient – how much we laugh out loud. Adults tend to overthink laughter. It can be helpful to grant yourself permission to intentionally laugh. Choose to schedule laughter – begin your day lovingly laughing at yourself in the mirror. This will set your day to laughter. Seek other opportunities to laugh out loud, whether that's joining a Laughter Yoga club, chuckling through a funny movie or integrating laughter intervals into your day. (See chapter three.) This will help redirect the laughter from your head into your heart. Please also refer to 'The Laughter Effect in Practice' (p.207) for more tips on how to connect to your laughter-side.

another zebra. We stopped reaching for our cameras and looked elsewhere to get our dopamine hit. Our brains can get used to anything, and after a while it stops noticing things. The same applies to humour: after a period you stop laughing at the same jokes or stimuli. More about our humour response in the coming chapters.

The laugh line

Our laughter timeline – our laugh line – shifts and shapes largely according to what's going on in our life: internal moods, external influences. The issue is when periods of laughter stagnation go unnoticed. Only after a hearty bout of laughter does it dawn on you that it has been a long dry spell between laughs.

Everyone has their own laugh line according to their own life story. Here is mine:

LAUGHTER CODE

LL	Literally loads	**O**	Occasional
L	Lots	**S**	Stagnation

→ Primary school years LL
→ Secondary school years O L
→ Post-school gap year LL
→ Uni O L
→ Early career O
→ Marriage BC (before children) LL
→ Marriage AC (after children) S O L
→ Postgrad study and working part-time (with two kids under seven) O S O
→ Training and then practising as a Laughter Yoga facilitator LL

→ Academic career O L

→ Chronic illness and bowel cancer S O

→ Caregiving to elderly parents while simultaneously parenting my own children O

→ Present-day life in general LL, positively influenced by an intentional daily laughter practice

While this laugh line is rudimentary, it speaks volumes. Laughter is a chameleon, adapting to whatever else is going on in our lives.

SKETCH OUT YOUR LAUGH LINE

1. Grab a pen and piece of paper or an iPad, anything with which you can draw.

2. Draw your own laugh line.

3. What patterns can you see?

4. Identify a daily practice that will bring more laughter into your life and strengthen your laugh line. Laugh out loud when something funny happens, don't leave laughter lingering on the inside, 'power laugh' for ten-second bouts, or scroll for memes or videos that get your giggle on. Only you will know what's likely to reap laugh-out-loud moments.

How social we are is a critical factor in our laugh line, specifically the quality and quantity of conversations we're having. The late Robert Provine, a professor of neurobiology and psychology at the University of Maryland, found that laughter occurs thirty times more frequently in social rather than solitary situations.[5] Contrary to our belief that laughter is by and large generated by a class clown, comedian or practical joker, Provine's team discovered that only 10 to 20 per cent of the laughter episodes were caused by jokes. Common statements such as, 'It was nice meeting you, too' – hardly comedy gold – were far more likely to produce laughter.

We may feel happy and content when we're alone, but social interaction is spruced up by laughter. It's a conversational tool – or linguistic 'punctuation effect', accompanying even the least humorous of discussions. Laughter sends an inclusive signal for others to join in. In general, speakers laugh 46 per cent more frequently than listeners, with laughter at times replacing words.[6] For example, I received a recent 'guesstimate' by a prospective builder for new decking, but when the builder came to measure up, his quote was laughable – nearly twice as much as he'd indicated it would be in our call. 'Ha ha,' I blurted out when he told me. 'I thought you said it would be half that amount, ha ha ha.' Conversational laughter ushered in an undertone of lightheartedness, filling awkward pauses, of which there were several. It also minimised the risk of the conversation veering in a hostile direction. Needless to say, based on his quote, he didn't get the job.

Laughter and relationships

Not only does laughter lubricate a conversation, but it also provides important reproductive and survival advantages, signalling safety, eliciting playfulness and regulating stress and negative arousal.[7] When it comes to considering a partner, a good sense of humour is consistently at the top of the 'must have' pile. Prior to online dating apps, in 1996, Provine analysed 3745 personal ads placed in eight local newspapers to see how important a sense of humour or laughter was for people seeking a mate. Females were 62 per cent more likely to mention laughter in their ads and were more likely to seek out a sense of humour, while men were more likely to offer it.[7]

And in the battle of the sexes, who wins for most laughs?

Men and women both laugh a lot, but females laugh more.[8] Provine's research found that in cross-gender conversations females laughed 126 per cent more than their male counterparts. Other research found the more a woman laughed aloud during first-time spontaneous encounters, the greater her self-reported interest in the man she was talking to. Men were more interested in women who laughed heartily in their presence.[9] Like out of a David Attenborough documentary, it appears a critical mating ritual is for the female to parade her laughter feathers to ensnare her mate. A ritualistic laughter dance where a partner cues more laugh moves before they make their move.

Studies have found that men's laughter is more contagious. When men laugh, they are 1.73 times more likely to make their partner laugh.[10] While to date there is no equivalent data on same-sex couples, an inference can be made that one partner will be the chief laughter instigator.

But how does the Laughter Effect play out over the course of a relationship? Do couples who laugh together stay together? According to Laura Kurtz, a social psychologist from the University of North Carolina, 'in general, couples who laugh more together tend to have higher-quality relationships'.[11] A principle that applies to any intimate relationship. Intuitively, it makes sense that laughing together (not at one another) is a supportive activity. It's a subject close to my heart, having invested over thirty years of extensive research into this question. Without a shadow of doubt, I have concluded it most certainly helps! I'm sure my lead participant, my husband, Danny, agrees.

Pockets of conflict arise in even the most compatible of partnerships, though. I recall years ago *we* decided to renovate our home. A four-to-six-month project that ballooned into over nine months. During this period, Danny was absent for chunks of time, shooting a documentary on the other side of the world. Each time he'd return home querying why something either was, or was not, a certain way. To which I'd calmy (inwardly swearing) respond: 'I asked your opinion and you said something along the lines of that you weren't in the right headspace to give it any thought, or that you didn't care, whatever I decided.'

On the face of it – fabulous. Full autonomy to me, with one caveat. Renovating and design are not really my thing. Thus began arduous months of inevitable dramas: differences of opinion with a defensive builder, and the not-so-inevitable: the decision to engage a certain cabinet-maker. Said cabinet-maker rocked up adorned with neck tattoos and high-ankle gangster-style runners. I joked with the family about his gangster vibes, safe in the knowledge that he hailed from trustworthy stock – his sweet elderly dad had built the kitchen cabinetry in our previous house. Sadly, my jesting proved more prophetic than amusing. His high runners turned out to be not only a fashion accessory but also a means to cleverly conceal his ankle monitors, courtesy not of the Adidas outlet but a correctional facility. He squirrelled away our kitchen deposit, which according to police enabled his sweet elderly papa to retire in style in his former home – in Greece. And as for me, aside from the financial blow, it also meant additional months of washing dishes in cold water *en plein air* in the middle of winter.

Burnout was nigh when Danny returned home from yet another filming jaunt. His opening remarks were the last straw.

'Why are the light fittings where they are?'

I was tempted to march him out the back door, close the door behind him and change the locks. A hastily, ill-formed thought. While the front door was an actual door, not even the most ingenious locksmith could construct a lock for a yet-to-exist back door. I held it together long enough for jet lag to overcome him and his head to hit the pillow. I knew the boys would be super excited to see him on their return and didn't want my sour mood to dampen the reunion. I left the house and pounded the pavement to restore calm, stopping to sit under the expanse of a tree in a nearby park. Still not ready to face his barrage of 'why's', I sifted through a repository of memories on my phone searching for the perfect choice to sway my frustration and welcome endearment to my *worse* half. Among the zillions of photos of the boys sticking out their tongues and pulling faces, I found a holiday snap from a short escape to Noumea, sans kids, mocktail in hand, lost in laughter. Reliving these fun memories tilted my mood away from the relational building wreck. Happy memories intact, I was eager to return home.

My decision to lose myself in these memories was a wise choice. Research finds that reminiscing about shared laughter has a positive influence on relationships, with greater benefits than generalised reminiscing.[12] Jennifer Aaker from the Stanford Graduate School of Business found that couples prompted to recall stories when they laughed together versus just happy moments reported being 20 per cent more satisfied in relationships. Sharing a smile or a giggle with your partner can break tension, create a sense of closeness and improve communication. Initially my reminiscing was one-sided, but it wasn't long before I could make light of what had transpired with Danny, joking how we'd make brilliant property flippers – a shoo-in for *Grand Designs*. When there's a difference of opinion, laughter offers a way to renovate relationships.

It also helps if you're funny, which works well for me, as I'm definitely the funnier one in our relationship. Just ask my reflection. Although, of course, it's not a competition. According to University of Kansas's associate professor of communication studies, Jeffrey Hall, 'It's good to have humour. It's better to see it in your partner. And it's best to share it.' That's what affirms your relationship. Even more important are the moments when you are both laughing together. Whether you're laughing at *The Bachelorette*, *Fawlty Towers* or *The Office*, sharing a common sense of humour is what counts. It's a relationship 'thrival' skill, making us feel safe within each other's company, conveying fun and playfulness – and we all know where that can lead ...

To infectious laughter, of course. It is believed Homo sapiens are the only species to engage in contagious laughter, possibly explaining why for centuries the Church and other institutions were anti-laughers, aligned with its view about sexual passion. If you can't control it, it can't be good. Laughter is contagious particularly at an earlier age. I'm sure there's a time in your younger life when you 'lost it', typically at an inappropriate moment.

I recall one such occasion as clear as day. My bat mitzvah, my entry into womanhood. For months, I'd excitedly prepared to lead my community in prayer for the first time in my own right. Filled with pride I confidently began reciting blessings, reading from the prayer book in my clearest projected voice. I proclaimed, 'Breast be ... .' instead of 'Blessed be ...' I knew I shouldn't have, but couldn't resist catching the eye of one of my friends to see if she'd noticed my blunder. Whether or not she had, the simple act of catching her attention propelled a laughter dart. I tried suppressing it. She tried suppressing it. Alas to no avail. It wasn't long before pockets of snickering erupted throughout the congregation. Thankfully the rabbi intervened, beckoning the community to join in the prayer while I composed myself, focusing my eyes on the prayer book and not a centimetre beyond. What a launch into womanhood. Breasts and all.

It's a well-known fact that laughter is contagious. That's why back in the 1950s, in the absence of a live audience, *The Hank McCune Show* revolutionised TV viewing by introducing the first laugh track. Ever since, laugh tracks have become a firm fixture in many sitcoms. Canned laughter may sound artificial, but it encourages TV viewers to laugh as if they were sitting in the crowd. I'd grown so accustomed to laugh tracks and live audience laughter that I'd failed to notice how integral they were to a show's vibe. That was until watching Shaun Micallef's *Mad as Hell* studio comedy show during the Covid pandemic. Not only was there no studio audience, but there was no substitute. Usually I'd be in hysterics, yet I strained to get a laugh out. I realised how much my laughter had been elicited by the laugh track.

You can induce your own laughter, too. Ask Freda Gonot-Schoupinsky from the University of Bolton in the UK. Responding to calls from the medical community for a practical laughter prescription, she developed the idea of the 'Laughie', to ensure people get at least one minute of daily laughter. The Laughie is similar to a selfie but instead of taking a photo of yourself, you record your own laughter for one minute using your phone. You then play back your recorded laughter, which prompts you to laugh. Her research found the Laughie elicited laughter for most of the one-minute duration in 89 per cent of the 420 Laughie trials; half of the participants found their laughter 'self-contagious', and many found it helpful.[13]

The more we laugh, the more we laugh. One of the most unbelievable accounts of a 'laughter contagion' comes from a girls' boarding school in Tanzania. It began in 1962, when three girls got the giggles and couldn't stop laughing. It quickly spread to ninety-five students, where uncontrollable laughter and intermittent crying bouts forced the school to close a couple of months later. But in that time the epidemic had spread further, with related outbreaks occurring in other schools and regions. Two and a half years later, nearly 1000 people had been afflicted. It has been said that the interminable laughter hysteria was, in part, related to the stress of becoming a new republic.

For a 'laughter contagion' to occur, it requires a person to not only hear laughter, but also to see laughter. This signals mirror neurons in the brain to fire. Seeing someone smile, for example, creates an association in your own mind with smiling. You don't even need to think about why this person is smiling. It's immediate and effortless.

ACTIVATE YOUR MIRROR NEURONS

Practise activating your mirror neurons. Choose a partner and sit opposite one another. Naturally begin a conversation but don't tell your partner it's a scientific experiment. Observe what happens physically. Are you beginning to mirror one another's movements? What happens if you add some smiling or laughter to the conversation? Does it become contagious? If so, that will be your mirror neurons, firing and wiring.

I have seen firsthand the Laughter Effect of mirror neurons. A few years ago, I was privileged to be part of a team that delivered a world-first Laughter Yoga research project for people receiving dialysis treatment in a major hospital in Melbourne. Stepping into the dialysis ward for the very first time, I was struck by how subdued it was. Eye contact, one of the critical aspects of the success of Laughter Yoga, was near impossible, as individual blood-filtering machines the size of old-fashioned computers obstructed patients' views of one another. One arm was hooked up to the dialysis machine, leaving the other free, but for some, they were coping with amputated limbs or other forms of disability associated with kidney disease. Not usually prone to doubting the therapeutic benefits of laughter, to say I was hesitant about the program's success would be an understatement.

Yet, supported by other laughter therapists and the exceptional nursing staff, in no time at all, light and laughter transformed the ward. At the conclusion of one of the sessions, I was curious to glean one gentleman's experience of Laughter Yoga. At the beginning of the program his eyes were dull and darkened, visibly weighed down by sadness. Though, afterwards, when I looked into his eyes, I observed a bright twinkly beam of light emanating from behind them. I assumed there to be a spotlight directed into his face. However, when I swivelled around, all I saw was the harsh standard hospital lighting. Despite still being hooked up to the dialysis machine, his mirror neurons were firing and wiring, visibly sparking joy and light.

The conversational and contagious properties of laughter help to explain why our twilight years are often characterised by less laughter. There are fewer opportunities to see and hear it. The laughter punctuation effect can only work when there's conversation to punctuate. You don't necessarily need to bring in the clowns, but simply scheduling opportunities for chitchat can reduce loneliness and social isolation, and increase possibilities for a chuckle. Having spent considerable time in residential care over the years, both in a personal and professional capacity, I have observed loneliness up close. However, I've also been introduced to amusing 'senior chat' vernacular, including BFF (Best Friend Fainted); BYOT (Bring Your Own Teeth); LMDO (Laughing My Dentures Out); GGPBL (Gotta Go, Pacemaker Battery Low).

Residential aged care was a path my mum was seemingly destined for. However, her decline from Alzheimer's was so swift, the move never transpired. Within the space of six or so weeks, she went from being lovingly tended to by my dad and a part-time carer in her home, to lapsing in and out of consciousness in hospital. We were advised her end was near and the decision was made for my US-based sister to return home. On Mother's Day, Mum had a lucid spell. It was, we thought, a Mother's Day miracle: she was defying medical odds and returning to us. It didn't last.

When my sister, Natalie, arrived, Mum was unconscious, presumably unaware that her daughter had travelled halfway around the world to be by her side. In her hurried and harried dash across the Pacific, Natalie bemoaned that she'd forgotten to pack a change of bra. 'That's a shame. You'll need all the support you can at this time,' I retorted. A second or two passed before the humour processing kicked in and the family, my bereft dad included, were all lost in laughter. To our shock and amazement, a gentle smile appeared on Mum's face. We will never know what pierced her unconsciousness: was it the humour stimulus or the contagious nature of laughter? Mum's response was a final blessing. Held in humour's embrace, here was an opportunity to defuse the sadness with tears of joy, release and relief.

. . . .

From the cradle to the grave, one spot on the globe to another, the Laughter Effect helps us thrive. We're wired to smile and laugh over a lifespan. It's a genetic imperative helping us bond and connect to our external world – enabling us to be more present with one another. As we age, our minds might forget but our bodies do not. A laugh-force anchoring us in the essence of joy, love and connection. As American essayist Agnes Repplier penned, 'We cannot really love anybody with whom we never laugh.' To this I add, we cannot really love ourselves if we never laugh.

DRAW YOUR LAUGHTER SELF

Time to get arty. You'll need a piece of card or paper that is small enough to carry with you. Connect to your laughter-side by doodling or drawing what it feels like to be immersed in laughter – a visual representation of your joy. You might like to draw yourself feeling on top of the world, how you feel after a good dose of laughter or simply fill your page with a colour or pattern that evokes happiness.

When you're done, you may like to put this image in your wallet or purse. You can then purposefully pull it out when you're in need of some mood-brightening. Or it might provide a joyful surprise when you accidentally stumble upon it. Alternatively, pop it on your fridge or have it on your desk . . . whatever will draw your attention to it. You might even like to take a photo of it and use it as a screensaver on your phone or computer.

It will serve as a conscious reminder of the positive flow of emotions elicited by your smiling or laughing self.

3

The Best Medicine

Always laugh when you can, it's cheap medicine

—Lord Byron

Where to begin in quantifying laughter as medicine? It's not as if it can be bottled and the contents analysed and measured in a lab. (Although baby test tubes of laughter would be cute!) That's not to say laughter research isn't being conducted. To the contrary, it's a burgeoning field. It's no surprise laughter research is growing in popularity, as the quest for a solution to our stressed-out modern lives continues. Pharmaceutical companies are competing to find a cure to this mounting twenty-first-century problem. Mental health–related medications were dispensed to 4.4 million Australians between July 2019 and June 2020, equating to 17.2 per cent of the population.[1] In the wake of the global pandemic, mental health has taken a battering. Thankfully, laughter offers a complementary approach.

Until the latter part of the twentieth century, the study of laughter largely belonged to the domain of philosophers and naturalists, with some notable exceptions. The adage *laughter is the best medicine* is believed to be attributed to Henri de Mondeville, surgeon to King Philip IV, in the 1300s. After performing surgery, de Mondeville reportedly told jokes.

He wrote at the time, 'Let the surgeon take care to regulate the whole regimen of the patient's life for joy and happiness allowing his relatives and special friends to cheer him and by having someone tell him jokes.' As much as I'm an advocate for all things laughter-related, I'm relieved that when I underwent major bowel surgery, my surgeon didn't embrace de Mondeville methods. I think his brand of laughter therapy was more medieval than remedial. Anaesthesia was still four centuries away!

It wasn't until Norman Cousins published *An Anatomy of an Illness* in 1979, based on his experiences using laughter to buy him pain-free time, that the medical establishment began to take laughter as a therapeutic option seriously.[2] As we've discussed, Cousins, who had ankylosing spondylitis, checked out of hospital, believing his condition would be hindered by the hospital environment – full of germs, infections and bacteria – and self-prescribed a diet of comedy. His book was the first documented case study of the healing power of laughter as therapy.

Early laughter research was exclusively humour-based. Non-humour-based laughter – intentional or simulated – only guffawed onto the scene in 1995 with the birth of Laughter Yoga in India.

As a therapy, laughter can be classified into five categories:

- genuine or spontaneous

- self-initiated or simulated

- stimulated (the additional 't' must be for tickling!)

- pathological (which occurs either in illness or often as a result of a brain injury)

- induced, through legal means (nitrous oxide, aka happy gas, or cannabis).

Whether spontaneous, simulated or stimulated, laughter is recognised by the repetitive vocalisation of *ho ho*, *ha ha* or *he he*. Most of the research that follows in this chapter focuses on spontaneous and simulated laughter, although there will be some discussion on tickling, aka stimulated laughter, a little later.

Spontaneous laughter

Let's begin our exploration with spontaneous laughter. That's the variety that responds to something funny happening and a humorous response kicking in, from comedic events, amusing videos, clowns or jokes. By way of example, one of my late dad's favourite jokes (note, he was a physician):

> Patient: 'Doctor, will I be able to play the piano after this procedure?'
> Doctor: 'I don't see why not.'
> Patient: 'That's amazing, because I couldn't before.'

Simulated laughter

Simulated laughter, on the other hand, does not rely on a humour stimulus to generate it. The laughter is initiated first in the body and then the mind follows. It is not dependent on positive or humorous feel-good emotions.

This non-humour-based, self-initiated laughter therapy, most commonly Laughter Yoga, involves simulated laughter exercises, together with clapping and intervals of pranayama deep breathing. It is typically done in groups. Our brain believes the laughter is real, with a caveat: laughter can't be under duress or forced, as in the 'you will laugh' variety. Simulated laughter may not stem from something funny happening, but in no time at all, particularly if conducted in groups, the Laughter Effect heralds a lot of amusement and joy.

The ultimate stress buster?

One of the most common research areas is investigating laughter's effect – humour or non-humour based – on stress, anxiety and depression. Stress, per se, is not the enemy. It's how we react or respond that can be problematic. Responding with levity acts as a railway track change: it switches off the flow of stress hormones and the fight-or-flight reflex – which causes epinephrine or adrenaline to be released by the brain and distributed throughout the body – and switches on beta endorphins, our body's internal source of morphine that transmits messages between neurons, dulling signals of physical pain and psychological stress.

Prominent humour researcher Professor Lee Berk noted that the biochemical changes during laughter are almost the exact opposite of what happens to a body under distress. It appears frequency, rather than intensity, has the most impactful stress-buffering effect on daily life. A Swiss study with forty-five college students used a specially designed app for smartphones, prompting participants randomly throughout their day to answer questions regarding the frequency or intensity of laughter. It also mapped stressful events and stress symptoms experienced since the last prompt. After three months, researchers found one or two hearty laughs could not compete with frequent *tee hee hees* in terms of stress reduction.[3]

Furthermore, in a community-based Japanese study, laughter was evaluated from three perspectives: frequency, opportunities and interpersonal interactions. It found that (after adjustment for depression, sociodemographic factors and social participation) men and women who never, or almost never, laughed experienced overall poorer subjective health. A higher daily frequency of laughter was associated with lower prevalence of cardiovascular diseases, for which stress is a known precursor, and less laughter associated with increased likelihood of cardiovascular disease.[4]

Simulated versus spontaneous laughter in the brain and body

Japanese researchers have identified different neural pathways involved in simulated and spontaneous laughter. They conducted neuroimaging of pleasant emotions of participants viewing comedy films and found different areas of the brain would light up when mimicking a smile/laugh as opposed to when it was spontaneous.[5]

And in a University of Auckland study, the cardiovascular effects of both spontaneous and simulated laughter were investigated.[6] A sample of seventy-two participants was randomised to one of three six-minute interventions. Participants in the simulated laughter condition were asked to generate fake (self-initiated) laughter; others viewed a humorous video in the spontaneous laughter group, and the control group watched a non-humorous documentary. This was followed by a laboratory stress task. Results found the cardiovascular benefit was more pronounced in simulated laughter, yet all resulted in a happy heart.

Another study demonstrated a significantly higher incidence of all-cause mortality and cardiovascular disease in participants who laughed less.[7] A heartening result demonstrating the link between *ha,ha,ha* and *aaah*, where there's a decrease in stress hormones and the body exhales.

Laughter and the immune system

Long-term stress results in the depletion of white blood cell reserves needed to fight off infection and disease. Multitudes of mirth help in the creation of new white blood cells to boost the immune system in a process known to increase spontaneous lymphocyte blastogenesis – something that sounds straight out of *Star Wars* – the natural killer (NK) cells that destroy tumours and viruses. Because of the role of NK cells in viral illness and various types of cancer, the ability to significantly increase NK cell activity in a brief period using a non-invasive method, such as laughter, has exciting potential.[8] Moreover, a disease-fighting protein – gamma interferon – produces disease-destroying antibodies and T-cells, with effects lasting for twelve hours after the humour intervention. The more laughter flows, the better the lymph flow, helping transport fluids back to blood which defends the body against disease. In layman's terms, LOL-ing balances all components of the immune system, helping us fight off illness.[9] It also provides a workout for our vagus nerve, which runs from our brain to our gut and acts as a two-way super messaging highway that activates our parasympathetic nervous system, so we feel calmer and more at peace. This is known as *eustress* – positive stress, which relates to a stressful situation that we feel we're able to handle, and therefore results in a positive response with beneficial health outcomes.

A healthy high and humour in pain relief

Endorphins, our brain's feel-good neurotransmitters, boost feelings of pleasure, minimise perception of pain and create a temporary yet powerful sense of wellbeing. Laughter increases pleasurable sensations and triggers endorphins.[10] A range of studies have investigated pain tolerance after a good chuckle. Even in children.[11] One study involved showing children (aged between seven and sixteen) humorous movies before, during and after placing a hand in cold water. Submersion time was recorded and examined in relation to how funny the children rated the movie. Children viewing the movie while their hand was in water felt less pain than those who were not watching a funny film. It's no surprise, then, clown doctors are so popular in paediatric wards, using humour to distract children and adolescents, and their caregivers, from the stress associated with a hospital stay.

In another study, conducted by James Rotton, PhD, from Florida International University, orthopaedic surgery patients who watched comedy movies requested fewer aspirin and tranquillisers than the group that viewed dramas. No doubt their funny bones were stimulated.

And in a University of Oxford study lab experiment, *Mr Bean* was put to the test. Could wit decrease pain or merely create a muddle? In part one of the study, resistance to mild pain was monitored as volunteers viewed clips from *Mr Bean* or *Friends*, or non-humorous shows, such as golf or wildlife programs. Pain in the form of a frozen wine-cooler sleeve was slipped onto the arm or from a blood-pressure cuff and pumped to the threshold of tolerance.[12] The real pain, I'm sure, was the realisation that wine would not be imbibed as part of the study. Part two of the study was conducted at the Edinburgh Fringe Festival. Volunteers watched either a stand-up comedy show or a theatrical drama. They were asked to lean against the wall with their legs at right angles, as if sitting on a straight-backed chair, both before and immediately after the performance. If you haven't done this before, I speak from personal experience: it can get a little uncomfortable for the old thighs. The study found just fifteen minutes of laughter increased the level of pain tolerance by around 10 per cent as endorphins were released. However, it wasn't good enough to laugh on the inside; endorphins kicked in most dramatically when participants laughed out loud. In the lab experiments, the neutral, non-humorous programming had no pain-alleviating effect whatsoever. Nor did watching drama at the Fringe Festival. This confirms two of my long-held beliefs: golf is far from amusing, and, when given the option, opt for the Edinburgh Comedy Festival over the Fringe Festival.

Endorphin release is an involuntary response, cued by repeated muscular exertion stemming from exhaling without drawing a breath. It makes sense they go into freefall when we're laughing. You may wonder why? Have you ever laughed without breathing? I have yet to meet anyone who has. As a repetitive muscular exertion, laughter provides a gentle aerobic workout. How does your body feel after a prolonged bout of laughter? Tired tummy muscles, sore jaws, gasping for air? When it comes to pain reduction, the more laughter the merrier, unless the root of your pain is abdominal or dental – ouch!

Get fit by laughing

For all those fitness junkies out there, have you ever thought about engaging in a laughter workout? You'll save heaps of money on a gym membership. The more you laugh, the more you breathe. Which means greater oxygenation in the blood, increasing oxygenation to the brain and body, and reducing pain and muscle tension. It provides a joyful breathwork practice, toning the diaphragm and respiratory system, as well as abdominal and facial muscles.

Not sure if you believe me? Think about something funny or laugh for no specific reason and set your timer for sixty seconds. Approximately 120 *ha, ha, ha* laughs. Not only will your facial muscles feel it, so will your abs.

The founder of gelotology, the late William Fry, said, 'laughter dips down into your lungs and just cleans them out'. When people laugh, they exhale more stale air than a normal breath from their lungs, including residual carbon dioxide. Unless you're prone to asthma, the more splutter the better. That's because laughter increases the concentration of salivary immunoglobulin A. Increased saliva production helps to defend against infectious organisms entering through the respiratory tract, and also may lead to coughing, helping to clear it of mucus (remember to cover your mouth so as not to shower others in your gloopy germs).

Laugh away calories

Weight loss is a serious business. In 2021 in Australia alone, the market size of the weight loss services industry was valued at a whopping $458 million! This figure is exclusive of gyms, personal trainers and exercise-oriented companies.

Research conducted by Vanderbilt University Medical Center

revealed laughing for ten to fifteen minutes burns between ten and forty calories.[13] That's because laughter increases your heart rate by 10 to 20 per cent. When you laugh, your metabolism increases as well, so even once you've stopped laughing, you'll burn more calories at rest. Over the course of a laughter-filled year, the daily calories burnt from laughing may result in a net loss of approximately 1.8 kilograms. If you really want to slim down, laugh it up!

LAUGHTER INTERVAL TRAINING

Time to conduct a little scientific experiment to observe what, if any, mental, emotional or physical changes occur after you've partaken in a laughter interval exercise.

You may have heard about the health benefits of interval training. Well, laughter interval training replaces another physical activity, such as running, with, you guessed it, laughter. If at any time during this training you start feeling dizzy or wheezy, please return to normal breathing.

1. Before you begin, make a mental note of how you feel. Are you tired, anxious or feeling calm? What about your body temperature? Are you hot, cold or just right like Goldilocks? How quickly is your heart beating? How are you feeling within yourself?

2. Set a timer for ten seconds. Take a deep breath in and then laugh out loud as hard as you possibly can. Now breathe deeply for ten seconds.

3. Take another deep breath in and then laugh out loud for twenty seconds. (Doesn't seem like much until you're hastening the countdown to zero.) Now twenty seconds of deep breathing – in and then out.

4. Ready for one final round? Set your timer for ten seconds and laugh as hard as you can. And now breathe for ten seconds. Congratulations, you've completed one full set of laughter intervals. Ready for the next?

5. Did you experience any mental, emotional or physical changes?

If this practice reaped positive rewards, imagine how you'd feel if you included even as little as one moment of dedicated laughter each day?

Do this power laugh, stress-busting practice when you feel the need. Aside from being a brilliant mental health booster, it's also a powerful aerobic workout!

Gerontology gelotology

As a gentle aerobic workout, laughter therapy is perfectly suited to a more sedentary lifestyle or older demographic. Sudoku, move over. A humour-based study from Loma Linda University in the United States reported decreased cortisol in older adults, resulting in improved short-term memory, as well as improvements in sleep quality and mood, increased life satisfaction and decreased pain.[14]

Twilight years dish up grief, sadness, declining mental and/or physical health, and mushy peas. Social isolation is rife, even in aged care facilities. That's not to say this affects all older people – some are blessed with good health and are able to laugh in their own home with loved ones until the end of their days. Though, sadly, that's the exception rather than the rule.

To help remedy this, specialists in the field are putting the Laughter Effect into practice, with roles such as Elder Clowns, Laughter Yogis and

Laughter Bosses. Canadian researchers found that clowns working in aged and dementia care may help increase the quality of life for seniors, their families and healthcare staff who work with them by connecting to the 'laughter scent' – bringing back long-forgotten memories, improving cognitive functioning and communication skills.[15] In the Sydney Multi-site Intervention of Laughter Bosses and Elder Clowns study (SMILE), aged care staff were trained as Laughter Bosses, working alongside professional humour therapists, Elder Clowns.[16] The study found that residents who experienced a higher dose of humour and engagement experienced lower levels of depression. There was also improvement in social engagement and self-rated quality of life, and a reduction in behavioural disturbances and agitation.

A former colleague of mine from La Trobe University, Dr Julie Ellis, and I put this to the test, introducing The Laugh out Loud (LOL) pilot project in residential aged care.[17] Over a period of six weeks, in multiple aged care facilities across Victoria, we conducted thirty-minute Laughter Yoga sessions with groups of eight to twelve residents, once a week. Each week we ran the exact same routine, beginning and concluding with blood pressure measurement. We also investigated positive and negative affect and happiness levels using self-report questionnaires.[18] Residents unable to answer questionnaires by themselves were assisted by staff. I'll never forget the quizzical look on an early career nurse tasked with taking residents' blood pressure (BP) after our first session. Measurements before the session and after the session were quite different: most residents' post-session BPs were markedly down. I explained that, as happens with other aerobic activities, BPs initially go up, and then as the body eases into the exercise it goes back down. The nurse was relieved.

Results of our research also indicated an increase in participants' positive mood and pleasurable engagement with their environment. There was more enthusiasm and alertness, decreased lethargy and sadness, and an overall increase in the average happiness score.[19] I didn't need to wait for the results to confirm what my heart felt and my eyes saw. Frequently, after sessions, residents embraced me, asking when I'd be coming again and thanking me for helping them laugh. Tears of sadness were exchanged for tears of joy. Laughter wasn't only good medicine for the body; it raised spirits and touched their souls.

In Colombia, a laughter therapy program performed by Hospital Clowns for residents in aged care investigated the Laughter Effect on depression and loneliness. It found significant decreases in depression, although no significant changes in loneliness levels. This highlights an important distinction between depression and loneliness. Despite laughter's favourable effect on social relationships and its ability to lessen symptoms of depression, not even laughter can fill all voids.[20]

Two Iranian studies on elderly depressed women found Laughter Yoga to be at least as effective as a group exercise program in improving depression and life satisfaction.[21] Both therapies, acting as a form of aerobic exercise, were beneficial; however, when it came to improving life satisfaction, the Laughter Yoga group demonstrated greater increases than the control group. In another study, retired women received Laughter Yoga twice weekly for eight weeks, while the control group kept on with their routine daily activities. Results showed significant differences in the pattern of depression and anxiety scores within and between the Laughter Yoga intervention and the control group.[22] Anxiety scores increased in the control group, while notably decreased in the Laughter Yoga intervention group. And from week four, the Laughter Yoga intervention average depression scores were statistically lower than the control group.

When it comes to choosing between methods to alleviate depression and anxiety, research suggests choosing non-humorous over humorous therapies. No joke – they have been shown to be twice as effective.[23]

The 'un–Laughter Effect'

What if we turned this hypothesis on its head? Can a reduction of laughter frequency cause symptoms of depression? The 'un-Laughter Effect'.

Limited laughter was one of the hypotheses tested in the Deakin University–led dialysis research study I was part of.[24] Statistically, people on dialysis have one of the highest disability-adjusted life years of any chronic illness. Kidneys are critical for ridding the body of toxins. When they give up or are impaired, a range of complex health issues can arise. If the body can't naturally detox, dialysis treatment is required. Three times a week for up to five hours at a time, the patient is hooked up to a blood-filtering machine. A life sentence. Opportunities for travel are limited to places that have dialysis units on hand, which impacts socialising and makes full-time work problematic. It's no wonder depression is common.

One of the rationales for choosing non-humour laughter therapy is that it doesn't rely on a funny situation for laughter to occur. Over a four-week period, three times a week, thirty-minute structured Laughter Yoga sessions were conducted at Monash Health public hospital. Quality of life, subjective (self-reported) wellbeing, blood pressure, muscle cramping and lung function were measured.

Peals of laughter ricocheted around the hospital ward. Passers-by frequently popped their heads in, wondering what the hell was going on. Nurses, doctors and patients were lost in laughter. Everyone wanted a part of the laughter action. The feel-good vibes were contagious, the only desirable contagion in any hospital ward. Patients were literally laughing themselves towards happiness, as the research revealed. Stimulating the production of feel-good neurochemicals, such as endorphins and dopamine, elevated wellbeing and promoted calm.

Jocularity to reduce the jitters

There is nothing better than a good belly laugh to relieve nervous jitters and butterflies. Twelve months after my bowel resection, I had a review CT scan to make sure everything was in tip-top shape. My colorectal specialist reported that everything looked good aside from a liver spot, which he didn't think was previously there. Liver spot – what? My heart sank as a follow-up appointment was recommended with my gastroenterologist, who glanced at the scan and said he thought it looked fine. The very same gastroenterologist who'd reassured me the polyp he'd removed in my rectum looked fine, so I wasn't convinced. He recommended an MRI, just to make sure, although suggested I hold off for three months given the amount of radiation I'd been exposed to in the year my life took a detour. He reassured me and told me not to worry too much. As well-intended as these sentiments may have been, they did little to quell my fluttering heart and anxiety, which grew day by day, week by week, month by month. It was an inconvenient elephant in the room I was praying would not begin a stampede.

As much as I tried to shove them to the back of my mind, the past year's traumatic memories flooded my system. Two practices lessened my fear and heightened control of my emotional state: intentional laughter and deep breathing. When I was driving solo and stopped at traffic lights, I would laugh out loud until they changed to green. Anyone looking at me would have assumed I was laughing with a best friend, chatting hands-free on my phone. As part of my daily meditation practice, I added a spurt of laughter. The more I laughed out loud regularly, the less I felt the strangulating anxiety. My nerves weren't entirely gone – they didn't disappear until a little later after I received the 'all clear', thankfully – but the elephant stampede was certainly restrained.

FEEL LAUGHTER, NOT STRESS, IN YOUR BODY

1.   Place one hand gently around your throat and giggle a little
      he, he, he. Can you feel the vibration?

2.   Now, replenish your oxygen by breathing in and send your
      laughter deeper down into your chest. Place one hand on your
      chest and *ha, ha, ha.* Can you feel the laughter in your chest?

3.   Finally, send this laughter even deeper within, down to your
      belly. Place two hands on your belly as you inhale and then *ho,
      ho, ho* as you exhale laughter.

4.   Repeat this a few times and practise whenever you feel
      overcome by stress.

Chronic illness takes its toll, physically, emotionally and mentally. My experience of intermittent anxiety mirrors research results found in others facing chronic health issues, including cancer. A Korean study conducted laughter therapy with breast cancer patients: laughing in rhythm with clapping, laughing for a long time, laughing with the whole body, and laughing together with dance routines. A little cha, cha, cha with the *ha, ha, ha.* Laughter was shown to be effective in reducing stress, depression and anxiety – and this was visible after only one session.[25] This study highlights a challenge gelotologists face: drawing overall conclusions about the Laughter Effect when so many different methods are used.

A gutful of laughter

Anxiety is an untamed beast. As much as it begins with thoughts in your head, it's a whole-body experience. It depletes serotonin, an important player in controlling mood, emotions, appetite and digestion. We have more serotonin receptors in our gut than in our head, which means anxiety and depression are common side effects of irritable bowel syndrome (IBS). An Iranian study found that a good belly laugh is good for the belly, with Laughter Yoga found to be more effective than anti-anxiety medication in reducing gastrointestinal symptoms.[26]

The laughter genie

Not only can a good chuckle transform a glum gut by stimulating neurotransmitters associated with wellbeing, but it can even change genes.[27] A study in Japan explored the effect that state of mind has on diabetes in two groups of participants with insulin-dependent type 2 diabetes. One group had blood glucose levels checked before and after viewing a really boring sixty-minute lecture, while the other (luckier) group viewed an hour of comedy. The laughter group showed a significant drop in the need to top up with insulin, compared with the other group.

It gets even better. Researchers discovered twenty-three gene expressions had been altered just by laughing! It is believed the participants' elevated mood triggered their brains to send new signals to cells, which turned on genetic variations that allowed for a natural regulation of blood sugar.

Speaking of genes, laughter frequency has been shown to be an important factor in females wanting to get pregnant. A study involving women receiving IVF in Israel found 36 per cent of participants who were exposed to a medical clown for fifteen minutes after the procedure became pregnant, versus only 20 per cent for the comedy-free embryo.[28] So, if you're trying to get pregnant, why not enjoy a productive laugh together. Worst-case scenario: you'll have a laugh. Best-case scenario: you'll have a life!

From tired to recharged

Fatigue is debilitating. It's a sensation I'm all too familiar with, having had chronic fatigue syndrome in my twenties. Trying to combat fatigue was also one of the reasons I pursued Laughter Yoga. I felt enlivened after my first Laughter Yoga experience. No surprise then that when a health-promotion honours student at La Trobe University approached me to supervise a Laughter Yoga project measuring stress, anxiety and fatigue, I was elated. Bleary-eyed, stressed-out students were a sight I'd get used to, especially towards the year's end. In the four weeks leading up to end-of-year exams, we conducted weekly forty-minute Laughter Yoga sessions with ten to twelve students. Each week surveys relating to stress, anxiety and fatigue were completed before and after the session. Many students remarked on how their sleep improved a night or two after the session. They expressed improved motivation to study and overall enhanced mental clarity. Positive wellbeing increased and psychological distress and fatigue decreased. The honours student, who'd worked diligently planning, programming, implementing and later evaluating the project, was delighted.

How laughter changes your brain

As Danish-American comedian Victor Borge famously remarked, 'laughter is the shortest distance between two people'. Laughter, as we've explored, fills uncomfortable silences or mildly awkward encounters with its punctuation effect. But did you know putting on your metaphorical laughter lenses can literally change the way you see the world? Australian neuroscientist Professor Jack Pettigrew was investigating how the brain processes optical illusions and found a by-product of a good laugh is that it alters how a person perceives a drawn figure.[29] A Necker cube – an optical illusion involving a simple wire-frame drawing of a cube – was used in his experiment. He was telling a joke to one of his research participants when he made his discovery by accident. One can only hazard a guess as to what this neuroscientist's joke might have been. Perhaps:

Q: Why didn't the brain want to take a bath?
A: Because it didn't want to be brainwashed.

Back to the brainy stuff, when it comes to optical illusions like the Necker cube our perception shifts, enabling us to simultaneously see the cube from two different angles. Pettigrew discovered that during laughter, the brain blends the images together so that the illusion is lost and only a two-dimensional drawing is seen. He concluded: 'If you see both versions together, you can be pretty sure you're seeing from both hemispheres at the same time.' In science speak, 'laughter abolishes binocular rivalry', meaning that our perception seamlessly blends different images presented to each eye. Laughter modifies our brain state, changing our perception. Try it out yourself. Draw a Necker cube on a piece of paper, or if you're at a party and looking to impress, sketch it on a serviette. Ask someone to look at it then tell them a joke. See what happens.

Researchers using an MRI studied the brain during joyous laughter. In people who laughed at something humorous, gamma waves were produced in both hemispheres of the brain. Laughter, or simply enjoying some humour, increased the release of endorphins and dopamine in the brain, providing a sense of pleasure and reward. Higher levels of these uplifting hormones increased brainwave activity, specifically neural oscillations. Essentially, it exercised the entire brain. Professor Lee Berk called it 'being in the zone'.[30] The Laughter Effect immediately produces the same brainwave frequencies experienced by people in a true meditative state.

Laughter and longevity

Now to the burning question. Is the secret to a longer life more laughter? Looks like we're in with a good chance. A study of Latin American and white European mothers found that despite socioeconomic and psychosocial disadvantage of Latinos in the United States, they had greater life expectancy than other groups. It found that Latin American mothers laugh more than white European mothers, mediated by substantive conversations with others, resulting in what is known as 'The Latinx Health Paradox'.[31] Latin American mums' conversational prowess resulted in more laughter. The research found that laughing less may be a factor in functional disability later in life. People who laugh less may have difficulties with daily living activities, such as grasping and fine manipulation of objects due to pain or immobility or motor problems, including difficulties with inserting a key into a lock, typing or even buttoning a shirt.[32]

The best medicine?

Laughter unlocks so many physical, emotional, social and spiritual benefits, yet is it plausible to conclude that it is the best medicine? The science of laughter as medicine is a relatively new and emerging field of research. There is a need for more studies that use the same laughter formula. Including a control group would allow for greater ease in separating the laughter from other strands; for example, cha, cha, cha from *ha, ha, ha* – a standard physical workout versus a laughter workout. Different methods and study designs make comparing laughter apples with laughter apples a little unreliable – at times they're more like a funny fruit salad.

However, laughter therapies are certainly medically beneficial, and well suited to people at any stage of life and ability. Non-humorous laughter is particularly well suited to older people or those cognitively impaired, not relying on verbal skills such as wordplay or intellectual humour. It's safe for most people to try and is a joyful complementary intervention. As with any medication, it needs to be dosed correctly. One *ha* will hardly save a life.

Technology may provide the solution for more definitive answers on the therapeutic effectiveness of the Laughter Effect to help discern whether the suggested positive effects of the therapies are mediated by laughter itself, or something else. Smartphones could measure laughter using facial recognition and voice analysis. Or another kind of fancy device, a diaphragm electromyogram, could provide an exact measurement of laughter by assessing respiratory drive and diaphragm function.[33] This would assist in establishing the recommended minimal daily 'dosage', which at present is at least fifteen minutes, drip-fed throughout the day or in one exhaustive go.

For cynics who don't believe laughter can be prescribed – it can. There is already a social prescription, when health professionals refer patients to non-clinical services in the community for health-promoting activities, including gardening, (healthy) cooking classes, volunteering, art activities, adult learning or sports. And now an expansion of the social prescription to include a laughter prescription is endorsed by some within the medical community,[34] where people are directed to online or face-to-face laughter groups – most commonly, Laughter Yoga – to commune with others and dose up on laughter. Here is a laughter prescription by Laughter yogi and wellbeing educator Janni Goss, author of *Love, Laughter and Longevity*:

Share your smile.

Avoid bad news. Look for good news.

Play, laugh and have fun with the people in your life, especially children.

Access more comedy – TV, movies, radio, podcasts, internet.

Be an optimist – have hope in your life.

Exercise your sense of humour.

Use humour to de-stress. Laugh at yourself.

Find a laughter club and experience Laughter Yoga.

Seek help if laughter is elusive.

Give thanks for the benefits of laughter.

The health benefits of laughter can outweigh the efficacy of some pharmaceutical drugs – as proven by research and studies – much to the envy of the medical world. Perhaps if laughter was a more complex behaviour, many in the scientific community would be willing to accept the evidence of its success. Instead, they'd fight it out for the big laughter bucks. In the interim, who needs laughter in a pill when we've boundless supplies on tap. As one doctor remarked, 'If you boil a funny bone, it becomes a laughing-stock. That's pretty humerus.' The stronger the stock, the richer the health benefits. Let laughter be your medicine. As Dr Kataria said, 'There is no laughter in medicine, but there is lots of medicine in laughter.'

4

Laughter Yoga and Laughter Wellness

We don't laugh because we're happy, we are happy
because we laugh

—William James

Necessity is the mother of all inventions. Laughter Yoga and Laughter Wellness are examples of such, filling a void in the laughter therapy world. They involve inducing laughter through a structured formula of intentional laughter exercises, together with clapping and deep breathing exercises. Laughter Yoga facilitates health benefits for the body, mind and soul, especially during periods of adversity. You don't need to rely on something funny happening in order to reap the rewards. Laughter Yoga is one of the most enlightening activities you can choose to provide your daily wellbeing DOSE.

Intentional laughter involves reversing a lifetime of conditioning, as our logical mind initially kicks up a storm at laughing for no apparent reason. Yet through the power of neuroplasticity – the brain's ability to change itself – and with practice, in time a laughter mindset, a core component of the Laughter Effect, becomes hardwired.

As previously discussed, Laughter Yoga was conceived in the land of gurus – India, specifically in a park in Mumbai. Back in the 1990s, then editor of a health magazine, Dr Madan Kataria was seeking a solution to his growing stress levels and chose to write a feature about laughter being the best medicine. Though surprised at how much evidence there was to back up the claim, he was baffled by its nominal use in an everyday context. Research he found whet his appetite for a taste of this medicine. Loaded with jokes, Kataria went to his local park with five friends and began a 'laughter club'. After ten days, the joke supply was exhausted, not everyone was laughing and his friends wanted out. Refusing to give in, Kataria promised he would try to find a way to keep laughing without jokes.

One particular book, *The Complete Guide to Your Emotions and Your Health* by Emrika Padus, made a lasting impression on Kataria. His next step was informed by the book's key takeaway – your body cannot differentiate between whether you are really happy or if you are only acting like you're happy. Kataria consulted his wife, Madhuri, a seasoned yogi, who noted the similarity between laughter and yoga breathing exercises (pranayama). A formula was devised by Kataria – repetitions of breath; clapping; chanting *ho, ho, ha, ha, ha*; and assorted laughter exercises inspired by life rather than jokes or comedy – which would enable participants to choose to laugh rather than rely on chance.

Back in the park, the group started to 'fake' laugh for one minute using this new formula. Due to the infectious nature of laughter, they couldn't stop! The laughter exercise repertoire expanded, as did its following, and within five years Laughter Yoga had spread to fifty countries. It has become such a global phenomenon that it has its own dedicated day: World Laughter Day, celebrated on the first Sunday in May in over 100 countries. There are now thousands of Laughter Yoga clubs worldwide, with people coming together to laugh online and in person – one heart.

I'll be honest. I'm not a fan of 'fake it 'til you make it'. Fake, my friends, does not look good on anyone. My preference is 'make it 'til you make it'! This aligns with evidence that supports the brain's inability to distinguish between spontaneous and intentionally summoned actions. It also aligns to three power words: *Motion creates emotion*.

I'm sure there have been days where you have felt a tad glum. If you were to take yourself and this mood outside, you would be inclined to dawdle, head tilted down and shoulders slumped. Passers-by would likely avoid engagement – even a smile –assuming there's little point. The signal you are emitting is, *I'm feeling a little low, leave me alone.* What if you raised your head, expanded your chest to the sky, swung your arms more determinedly and picked up your pace? You'd send out a more upbeat vibe. Motion creates emotion: you have stomped your doldrums into the ground, leaving you more cheerful.

LET'S PUT IT TO THE TEST

1. Begin by clenching your fists, and in your own way embody stress.

2. Become aware of the positioning of your shoulders. Are they relaxed and soft or encroaching your ears? Has your breathing pattern softened or is it more laboured? In this stressful state, how are you feeling within yourself? Content? Stressed? Neutral?

3. Hold this sensation for ten or so seconds.

4. Now, exhale with a deep sigh. Allow your shoulders to relax and unclench your hands and fingers. With each exhale, release a little more stress. Release in whatever manner befits – deep exhales, stamping feet, shaking it out, smiling or laughing out loud. How are you feeling after a short amount of time? I would imagine a little lighter and brighter.

Modifying our physicality changes how we feel. Intentional laughter is no exception. Our body doesn't need to consult with our mind to *feel* laughter, whether it's spontaneous or simulated, and the type of stimulus doesn't matter. It could be a laughter exercise or a joke. That's why non-humour-based laughter is often referred to as a body-mind practice. Especially in instances where the mind thinks it doesn't feel like laughing, the feeling body can override the mind's false sense of superiority and let laughter loose. In no time at all, the mind takes a chill pill and, despite initial misgivings, disperses wellbeing chemicals throughout our body.

HERE ARE SOME SIMPLE GO-TO LAUGHS TO BEGIN YOUR INTENTIONAL LAUGHTER PRACTISE

1. Unzip your laughter

Pretend your mouth can be zipped up. With one hand unzip your mouth until it lets out zoodles of laughs. Unzip and rezip your laughter as many times as you'd like.

2. Mental floss

As we've explored, stress is one of the major reasons laughter shuts down. On a regular basis, just as you'd floss your teeth, pick up an imaginary string of mental floss and, laughing as you do so, tug from one ear to the other, clearing your mind of negativity and unwanted thoughts. When you're done, flick the floss away, with one final laugh.

Laughter Yoga is the primary model for non-humour-based laughter, though the Laughter Wellness method – devised by French-American Sebastien Gendry – builds on this. It too connects to the ancient wisdom of acting 'as if', where the body leads and the mind follows. It expands on the fundamentals of Laughter Yoga, offering a model to practise positive uplifting behaviours, and is comprised of four core elements:

- coordination movements, including clapping rhythmic activities, such as tapping on the thigh and the thymus point – located in the upper chest behind the breastbone – or brain gym exercises

- breathing, stretching and relaxing

- positive reinforcements to promote feeling good

- expressions of mirth (intentional laughter, song, dance or games).

The cognitive-behavioural therapies and self-care practices stretch not only people's smiles but also their experience of joy. They are designed to build trust, creativity, vitality, inspiration, compassion, communication skills and awareness, while promoting multiple aspects of wellbeing. If you're looking for a quick fix to boost positivity, Gendry is the first to admit that you're barking up the wrong tree. The path towards joy can be challenging: *some days I don't want to have to apologise, or face what I'm afraid of; I'd rather just complain, as opposed to taking a breath and deciding what comes next.* The Laughter Wellness method is a path to mindfulness, anchoring to the present moment with a smile, or your breath, enabling you to step outside of the past and future, and be more present. To acknowledge that happiness is not something you take, it's something you give yourself.

A LAUGHTER WELLNESS PRACTICE – FIND YOUR LAUGHTER

1. Close your eyes and be still.

2. Laugh on the inside, silently, without making a sound.

3. Hear your laughter on the inside. What does it sound like?

4. Breathe in and smile on each exhalation.

5. Keep your eyes closed. In your mind's eye, increase the volume of your laughter. Then, still with your eyes closed, laugh out loud.

You can also experiment with emitting different laughter sounds. Mouth closed or mouth open. Deep, belly laughter; shallow, chest laughter; or heady laughter. Whatever takes your fancy. Go where the laughter flows. Repeat as many times as you like until you feel more energised and joyful.

When you practise positive, uplifting behaviours and it feels good, this feeling begins to flow into your daily life. In Gendry's experience, it takes about ten minutes of physical engagement either for our mind, body or breath to shift. The breath is the linchpin between mind and body, working in synchronicity and mirroring one another. If you're stuck in your mind, you can break this circuit by breathing deeper or smiling. Initially the mind will resist. It will hound you to stop that behaviour, coming up with every excuse in the book – *You don't have time for this. What are you doing? You're being ridiculous.* However, if you engage and sustain the physical trigger, within ten minutes you'll create a shift in your biochemistry.

You can't simultaneously inhabit two opposing mindsets. When you're anchored in positive emotional states like laughter or smiling, you can't feel stressed or sad. This is one of the key tenets behind Laughter Yoga and Laughter Wellness, from which the Laughter Effect stems. It requires a behavioural shift so that desires like *I'd love to experience more joy in my life* don't remain in your mind. Transformation in your mind alone is a tough gig. Transforming in the presence of others can make it easier. Action is what separates the joy-makers from the joy-wannabes. 'Laughter works if you work it,' says Gendry, and he's right. Sending out a smile first changes yourself, then ripples out and changes how the world responds to you. Suddenly it's not such a scary, unfriendly place when everyone's smiling back at you.

Gendry expands on his methodology: 'It's not about being funny, it's about experiencing fun. It's not about forcing, it's about choosing to be. It's not about faking anything, it's about allowing yourself to experience a different way of being.' For Gendry, the impact has been profound. 'It hasn't changed my life, it has changed me.'

Can laughter bring world peace?

Embedded in the Laughter Yoga philosophy is the idea which Kataria espouses, 'When you laugh, you change and when you change, the world around you changes.' Integral to its mission is building global consciousness and friendship through laughter, enhancing health, happiness and, in the process, world peace. So not overly ambitious ;).

Laughter Yoga is changing lives in the least likely of places. Rwanda is a nation with a recent history racked by terror and trauma. In just 100 days in 1994, 70 per cent of the nation's Tutsi population, as well as moderate Hutus – approximately 800,000 people in total – were slaughtered by ethnic Hutu extremists. Victims were killed in their own villages or towns, many by their neighbours and fellow villagers. Decades on, families and friendships are still torn apart, and Rwanda remains in dire need of healing. Since 2010, West Australian Kim O'Meara – fittingly known as Angel Kimmy – has been spreading Laughter Yoga throughout Rwanda.

A little background on O'Meara. In 2000, she was diagnosed with CREST syndrome, a subtype of scleroderma. This condition, whose name means 'hardened skin', affects many internal organs and can become life-threatening. She was given three years to live. O'Meara describes her condition with great hilarity: 'The juices and elasticity are sucked out of your body, and you become a pigeon statue, where they can perch and poo on you, and eventually you become a fountain.' Responding to her diagnosis in a fashion few could ever mimic, O'Meara began laughing. She laughed about everything that had happened to her up until that moment, including being abused as a child. She laughed to a point many would deem inappropriate. Yet O'Meara is quick to point out there is always an appropriateness, a meaning in something: 'If you can laugh down to your belly about something other people can't even smile about, you can heal, you've got life down pat. Everything happens for a reason, everything is valid, all you have to do is to keep going until you find the funny side of it.'

Without laughter she is certain she would have died. A true optimist, she recounts a line from one of her favourite movies, *The Best Exotic Marigold Hotel*: 'If a story does not have a happy ending, it is not the ending yet,' adding, 'Stories go through drama, trauma, romance, comedy, and until you get to the part where the sum of these experiences is the joy of who you are, the expression of your life, then your story has not finished.' Despite CREST's visible mark on O'Meara's appearance, her spirit is far from crestfallen. She is the walking embodiment of living one's purpose in life despite, or perhaps because of, considerable disability.

Laughter Yoga introduced O'Meara to a practice for the laughter she had been voluntarily producing. In 2010, she packed her bags and set off for Rwanda with two missions in mind: she would hang out with gorillas, and she would explore introducing Laughter Yoga to this epicentre of trauma and torture. Inspired by Dr Kataria's vision to bring world peace through laughter, she believed that 'if you can do something there [Rwanda], you can do something anywhere'.

The first mission ended in a broken heart. One particular gorilla fell for O'Meara's alluring charms and was reportedly bereft at her departure. The second mission was far more successful, resulting in a partnership between the Western Australian Laughter Yoga Club in Perth and the Rwanda Resilience and Grounding organisation (RRGO), rehabilitating communities through Laughter Yoga. In one district, Bugesera, a Reconciliation village was created after the genocide, for victims and survivors to live alongside each other. Laughter Yoga was chosen by the Rwandan government as one of the rehabilitation techniques to be used as a way of attempting to make the country a peaceful place again, and asked RRGO to introduce the practice to the community. It's part of RRGO's broader mission to improve mental health and resilience in the Rwandan community by fostering positive emotions such as love, gratitude, kindness, optimism and forgiveness. Laughter Yoga training is combined with trauma therapy, drawing on O'Meara's art therapy background, working with clay to help process trauma. It has inspired the unimaginable: survivors laughing with those who tortured or killed their family. It's not diminishing peoples' trauma by insensitively laughing at it or condoning actions that may have caused the trauma; rather, it's working with laughter's endorphin effect. This enables participants to reach a 'loving' mental state where they can then view the atrocities they experienced from the height of laughter, instead of from a 'normal' emotional state, spiralling down.

The Rwandan government and independent researchers continue to monitor differences in mental wellbeing and resilience between perpetrators and victims. One regular Laughter Yoga participant said, 'I am feeling happy, peace, relaxed and I would like to bring this candle of peace in my family.' Rather than following a formula of laughter exercises popular elsewhere in the world, they've made the practice their own, creating culturally and lifestyle-appropriate exercises. An exercise using a mini straw broom to sweep the floor. And laughter accompanying the tradition of washing clothes with rocks. They even have a series of laughs involving unsuccessfully combing their curly hair, which according to O'Meara always guarantees uproarious chuckling.

A Rotary International grant in 2022 enabled the RRGO to begin Laughter Yoga training clubs in fifteen villages, with 230 trained facilitators and plans for a Laughter Yoga School. One of the laughter clubs is able to provide their village with milk and cheese, owing to O'Meara's resourcefulness. She raised funds and bought a pregnant cow – proclaiming a small victory, 'two for the price of one'. The laughter club is where residents come to laugh and drink milk together. 'Laughter is the most precious thing on the planet,' says O'Meara, whose grand vision is to have one minute of laughter included at the national genocide commemoration ceremony. The hope is that laughter will be what keeps people from fighting, preventing another genocide. A pathway to reconciliation, healing and peace building.

Laughter therapy is being used elsewhere in the world, in places with conflict and where tensions simmer to boiling point. Practitioner in the Art of Nonsense (seriously) and laughter therapy, Israeli Alex Sternick has conducted joint Laughter Yoga sessions for Israelis and Palestinians. Sternick stumbled upon Laughter Yoga while in India and was so inspired by Dr Kataria's message that 'laughter does not always solve a problem, but it helps dissolve one', he decided to import the practice into the long-running Middle East conflict. Sternick had heard of Sulhas, forgiveness festivals – the name is derived from the Arabic word *sulh*, meaning 'to make peace' or 'reconciliation'. So, sensitive to the complexities of bringing Jews and Palestinians together, in 2007 in Beit Jala – a neighbouring town of Bethlehem – Laughter Yoga was packaged into the two-day conflict-resolution workshop. Participants came from all over Israel and the Palestinian territories. In no time at all, labels and identities dissipated as a united collective of human beings, not warring individuals, shared laughter.

News travelled fast – to Jordan, from where Sternick received a request to remotely train a Jordanian woman in Laughter Yoga. After which, led by his newest recruit, the Laughter Effect rippled out to Syrian refugees. Peace, Sternick says, begins with the self. If you don't address your inner conflict, Laughter Yoga or any other technique can only go so far. 'When you're talking about external wars between people, it's because they have internal wars – personal problems or unresolved challenges – that causes them to hate others. So, if you don't work on these personal issues deeply and come to terms of peace with these parts [of yourself], you cannot really laugh with another person.' Sternick remarks, 'When you can be kind and accepting of yourself, you will stop hating others – it will evaporate.'

Connection between people in conflict with one another, he believes, needs to be non-verbal. 'It can be laughter, crying, gibberish, or even

SEROTONIN SISTER

I'm worried people will think I've lost my mind if I'm seen laughing for no reason.

I totally understand! If you're a self-conscious laugher, laugh in places you feel less vulnerable. The shower, home alone or in the car. Also, it can help to remind yourself why you're laughing – for the joy and health of it, the best reasons of all.

cooking a meal together. Then at least on some level the animosity begins to fade away.' Sternick observes that talk can sometimes exacerbate conflict. It separates people, but when you bring something from the body, such as laughter, it can lead to a one-on-one heart connection. Laughter Yoga enhances potential for deeper reconciliation – with the self and others.

It's a common thought shared in the humour domain outside the Laughter Yoga world, with many comedians recognising the power beyond 'just a laugh'. British comedian Alistair Barrie, who compered *Are You Taking the Peace?* – an irreverent stand-up show with a serious agenda – affirmed, 'The one way humanity has always coped with the horrors it surrounds itself with is by laughing at them, and that's at least something we all have in common.' Or, as UK-based Aussie comedian Adam Hills said, 'We wouldn't do what we did if we didn't think that what we were doing actually makes the world better. Which is a terrible thing to admit. But I think if you can unite a room in laughter, you've possibly one less division in the world.'

Laughter Yoga – the hard cell

Luis Gomez, counsellor and Laughter Yoga Master trainer, has a passion for facilitating Laughter Yoga in the penitentiary system in Mexico. When he began in 2013, there were over 40,000 prisoners in Mexico City alone, in thirteen prisons – two female and eleven male.[1] Spoilt for choice, Gomez started Laughter Yoga in female prisons, hoping it would be a softer landing, but he experienced teething problems. In one of the first sessions, the 'lion laugh' was acted out too literally when, sadly, some of the women became hostile and aggressive and bit their fellow prisoners. Thereafter, he pleaded with inmates to try to see the sessions as something positive that could really help them, and to come to the sessions with respect for each other.

Improvements in the way inmates related to one another during sessions gave him a lion's hunger for more. Together with prison psychologists and social workers, Gomez planned a twenty-two-day Laughter Yoga program in male prisons. He clearly does not shy from a challenge because rather than deliver the program to prisoners with some degree of freedom, he chose prisoners in solitary confinement to mix with each other for *Project Unleash Your Happiness*. Despite his small physical stature, Gomez felt safe and strong, empowered by his mission, saying, 'It's a matter of being aware, not afraid.' The program combined breathing exercises, Laughter Yoga exercises tailored to enhance rehabilitation and – wait for it – salsa!

Although met with resistance, Gomez simply said, 'Do what I am saying from the beginning to the end of the program and just see ...' It worked! Communication channels were opened. Hardened criminals, largely ostracised by society and starved of human contact, met one another up close and personal for the first time. Initially they were uncomfortable sharing a laugh, let alone a conversation, but in time they shared tears of laughter and tears of joy. Gomez believes that even when you're not incarcerated and have your freedom, you can still be a prisoner in your mind. He encouraged prisoners to shout, '*Soy libre!*' ('We are free!'). Despite the occasional retort of 'No you're not', ricocheting off the walls of a nearby cell, there was a shift. As one prisoner shared, 'For a few moments I felt like I was out of here.' Psychological tests, drawing activities and testimonies from family members astonished at their loved one's transformation, together with before and after 'mugshots' of a different kind, visibly demonstrated the program's success. Initial data has suggested lower recidivism rates in prisoners who share in the gift of laughter.

. . . .

On occasion we all feel trapped or powerless. Facing significant illness can be one such time – becoming a prisoner to your body. That's how I felt.

For many months, medical appointments, surgery and, later, recovery filled my days. My freedom was tempered. A laughter wellness mindset was instrumental to my healing. Had I solely relied on amusement or merriment to magically inspire positive emotional change, I would have waited a long time. Intentionally calling on the Laughter Effect promoted my empowerment and ability to thrive, not merely survive.

A laughter wellness mindset enabled me to embody the energy of positivity – through smiling and intentional laughter practices. And also through the written word, where I could challenge my inner (negative) voice. This is a practice we'll explore further in chapter ten. In doing so, I facilitated a mental, emotional and physical shift. First catalysing a change in my world, before extending it out into the external world.

LAUGHTER AFFIRMATIONS – 'LAFFIRMATIONS'

Here's one of my favourites:

> *I am love*
> *I am laughter*
> *I am joy*
> *I am peace*

Downward-facing 'black dog'

Sometimes laughter and its associated energy is so far removed it can feel like you may never experience it again. That's what it can be like for the many millions of people around the globe suffering from chronic anxiety or depression. Teetering on the brink, questioning the value of their life. Over the decades, I've met people who have admitted that Laughter Yoga saved their life – literally. As CEO of Laughter Yoga Australia, Merv

Neal, explains, 'It's a social communication response. When I'm laughing, I'm calling out to people that I'm having a good time.' Due to laughter's contagious energy, participants gain a mini respite from their despair. The more someone's day is filled with moments of laughter, even if cultivated from simulated laughter exercises, the greater the likelihood of raising spirits – even fleetingly. Greet yourself in the mirror each morning with a little giggle or laugh. Laugh to yourself in the shower. Our habits become our habitat, so build a laughter habitat.

BUDDY UP

Why leave laughter to chance? Find a work mate or friend and laugh for the health of it for a few minutes. Then build it up to five minutes. Phone your buddy, arrange a Zoom call or meet in person. Create a laughter habit. Struggling to find a laughter buddy? Be your own laughter buddy!

Feelings of low mood, depression and anxiety were especially prevalent during Covid-induced lockdowns around the world. Grief was real – for loved ones we were separated from and for the lives lost. Face-to-face social get-togethers with family and friends, hugs and bouts of side-splitting laughter were largely erased. In-person laughter clubs were one of the first casualties of a physically and socially distanced world, at a time when, more than ever, people were crying out for laughter.

Giving up wasn't an option, though the question on everyone's lips in the Laughter Yoga world was whether its effusive energy could translate online. Critical aspects of growing laughter momentum are eye contact and close physicality. Seeing laughter. Feeling laughter. After my first nerve-wracking virtual session, I cut out chanting and clapping as the dissonance and time lag was jarring, made the mute button my best friend, and, in a bid to create a communal feeling, insisted on gallery view and cameras on. I also stepped up intentional breathing practices to stimulate oxygenation after prolonged periods of being glued to a screen. Remarkably, after a few hitches, assimilation online was almost seamless. Laughter Yoga facilitators – myself included – tweaked their practice to one-dimensionality and a whole new breed of laughs was born, including the elbow bump greeting laugh and face mask laugh. Rather than signal Laughter Yoga's death knell, the pandemic enabled it to chime even louder and online groups popped up all over the globe.

I embraced the freedom that online sessions offered, enabling me to provide an *essential* service – laugh if you will – even in the middle of the rainforest. The universe had smiled kindly on me. I was on a yoga retreat in Far North Queensland when I received a request to facilitate a Laughter Yoga session for a customer service team locked down in Melbourne. Morale was at an all-time low as they responded to a rise in disgruntled clients, many of whom were experiencing financial hardships. Mindful of the disparities in our environments and not wanting to gloat, I briefly considered concealing my whereabouts. However, the rainforest's magnetic charm won over. I angled my laptop so that participants could soak up the magnificence of the rainforest scenery behind me. Echoes of laughter flowed out into the verdant horizon. The sky was the limit. After the session, which went down a treat, I bumped into retreat participants, many of whom knew me as the 'laughter lady'. They remarked on how the sound of laughter resounding through the rainforest lightened their mind and sparked a smile.

Laughter Yoga to brighten the sunset years

Whether it happens online, face to face or is carried by the breeze, the energy of laughter is heightened by aural and visual cues. This makes it an ideal wellbeing tool for when some of our senses might fade. The 'silver' generation have reason enough to mourn: long-lost love, loss of lifelong friends and, for those stepping over the threshold into residential aged care, loss of autonomy, relinquishing control over the beat of your day or perhaps farewelling a beloved pet. An aged care nurse shared a sad but not entirely surprising fact with me that anti-depressants are doled out to the majority of residents early in their transition. Overall, aged care staff do their best to raise spirits. However, to really impact wellbeing, particularly for individuals who have less to laugh about, laughter needs to be timetabled and not left to chance.

It's not solely about the laughter but where it might lead. Like your favourite tune, laughter acts as a 'trigger' to elicit the *do you remember when ... ?* moments. Those moments may have been a lifetime ago but reminiscing connects to laughter in the present moment. While the laughter may be ephemeral – all up, around ten to fifteen seconds – an unconscious mind shift is sustained through this gentle and joyful aerobic workout. Residents enter the room mirroring their age and leave under the youthful spell of laughter-sparkle dust.

I've seen play, something that underpins Laughter Yoga, rekindled in laughs such as the motorbike laugh (imagined bikes are revved to the rhythm of laughter). (One lady sassily revealed she'd ridden pillion as a twenty-something-year-old.) Gross motor skills and hand-eye coordination are stimulated by catching a smiley 'laughter' ball. Fine motor skills, activated by respectively tapping fingers back and forth, resulting in heightened dexterity and competency after only a few sessions in people who had suffered strokes. Vocal cords and playful cheekiness chords are stimulated by musical laughs, where *ha, ha, ha* replaces lyrics, although not always. On one occasion during a rendition of the song 'My Favourite Things' from *The Sound of Music*, one man deviated from *ha, ha, ha*, crooning about his favourite thing, SEX!

In many sessions I'd be struck by the potency of laughter. I witnessed feet tapping to the rhythm of *ho, ho, ha, ha, ha* in a somnolent wheelchair user. Someone with advanced dementia shared a moment of lucidity – smiling even if they didn't laugh out loud. Another was lost in slumber but joined in a laughter song's chorus. 'When will you be coming back?' was ringing in my ears after the final guffaw. Staff were keen to learn how they could make the practice their own and discovered they could diffuse *ho, ho, ha, ha, ha* throughout the day into exercise programs, art activities and gardening, calling upon the Laughter Effect to promote engagement and emotional and physical wellbeing in residents and staff, which flowed to loved ones. A daughter of one of my participants introduced herself, catching me off guard, and asked, 'What have you done to my mother?' To which I thought, *Shit, what have I done?* In actuality something wonderful, as the smile that had been absent from her mother's face for quite some time had been restored. It transpires you *can* teach an old dog new laughter tricks. Whether you're young or old, welcoming a new mindset or belief system doesn't happen overnight. It requires intention and practise until it becomes second nature. Or, more accurately, first nature, as the disposition to smile and laugh is, as we've explored, innate. Laughter Yoga and the Laughter Wellness method get us out of our heads and into our hearts.

Sometimes reassurance is needed to lessen internal resistance, giving ourselves permission to laugh, and to accept that it doesn't matter how the laugh started; our mind and body will feel very 'laughed'. If laughter is a short cut to happiness, intentional laughter is a means to get there. An interpersonal laugh skill raising our own vibration while deepening our connection to others.

If you haven't already done so, I encourage you to give Laughter Yoga a go. Online or in person. It might spell the beginning of something truly beautiful.

5

Our Sixth Sense – Humour

Humour is mankind's greatest blessing
—Mark Twain

You might think a sense of humour is simply something that determines your taste in jokes and what you find funny or not, but it's so much more than that. Humour stimulates multiple regions in our brain, where it's processed, and it deserves to be classified as our sixth sense. People who regularly exercise a sense of humour tend to live, love, lead and learn better. Hence why it's a core element of the Laughter Effect. And don't worry if you're not a natural comedian; like with all our senses, humour can be honed.

The term *humour* dates to assumptions made by Ancient Greek physicians that the human body is governed by four elemental liquids ('humours') that influence a person's health and temperament. Mirth is considered to be one of the elements.

Over centuries, the brightest of minds have attempted to understand the how and why of humour – but oh so seriously. Plato, Aristotle, Hobbes and Descartes believed humour was an expression of superiority. 'I think I am amused' equalled 'I think I am better than you.' When Darwin turned his mind to humour he was ridiculed for espousing that some animals – kookaburras and hyenas aside – laughed and even displayed a sense of humour. Images of Sigmund Freud, founder of psychoanalysis, might suggest solemnity, yet as a purveyor and connoisseur of funny jokes and stories, humour was one of his defining characteristics. Let's add Freud's Relief theory into the humour mix: laughter allows people to let off steam or release pent-up 'nervous energy'. Humour is a pressure valve for repressive psychic energy, which provides a mental break. Freud theorised that all wit and humour stemmed from the unconscious mind and that this was a healthy defence mechanism, reducing anxiety and emotional pain. Consistent with the lyrics written by 1970s Australian rock band Skyhooks, Freud agreed that 'ego' was a dirty word, believing individuals using humour to cope with challenges displayed a positively strong ego:

> Like jokes and the comic, humour has something liberating about it; but it also has something of grandeur and elevation, which is lacking in the other two ways of obtaining pleasure from intellectual activity ... the victorious assertion of the ego's invulnerability. The ego refuses to be distressed by the provocations of reality, to let it be compelled to suffer. It insists that it cannot be affected by the traumas of the external world; it shows, in fact, that such traumas are no more than occasions for it to gain pleasure.[1]

His theory contrasted with the Incongruity theory of humour, pioneered by philosophers Kant and Schopenhauer, which suggests humour arises when logic and familiarity are replaced by things that don't normally go together – such as a Hawaiian shirt with a tie. Here's another example.

A guy spots a sign outside a house that reads 'Talking Dog for Sale'. Intrigued, he walks in.

'So what have you done with your life?' he asks the dog.

'I've led a very full life,' says the dog. 'I lived in the Alps rescuing avalanche victims. Then I served my country in Iraq. And now I spend my days reading to the residents of a retirement home.'

The guy is flabbergasted. He asks the dog's owner, 'Why on earth would you want to get rid of an incredible dog like that?'

The owner says, 'Because he's a liar! He never did any of that!'

Whether you found the talking dog joke amusing or not isn't a reliable indicator of the health of your humerus. Not all incongruities are funny and not all humorous situations result in laughter. As we've established, laughter can arise from non-humorous situations. Generally, humour is identifiable by some form of behaviour: most commonly laughter and smiling with the occasional guffaw or snort. That's what discerns humour from amusement or enjoyment.

Despite many attempts to find a single unified theory about this sense, analysing humour is like trying to analyse love. It's hard to quantify. That certainly hasn't stopped quantum theorists from trying. Canadian and Australian researchers applied a mathematical framework in order to understand cognitive humour, which resulted in the Quantum Theory of Humour. It states that the probability of a joke being assessed as funny or not is proportional to the projection of the individual's understanding of the joke onto a basis representing funniness.[2] Don't know about you but I got lost at 'proportional'.

Humour is a highly sophisticated innate sense, a complex behaviour involving cognitive, emotional and motor responses. Once a stimulus is perceived as humorous, it will trigger a conscious or unconscious reaction resulting in a physiological (laughter), cognitive (wit) or emotional (mirth) response, or a combination of these.[3] To comprehend humour, the brain must complete two steps. The first involves being sensitive to the element of surprise in humour – that something unexpected has occurred. The second is going beyond the unexpected and looking for something that makes sense.

Neuroscientists have even discovered (by mistake) from where this sense stems. Investigating the cause of a young woman's severe epilepsy, they inserted an electrode into her skull. The more they prodded, the more she laughed. Rather than finding the root cause of her fits, they discovered

Comedy Central – the brain's laughter centre, a part of the brain called the cingulum bundle. Made up of white matter, this bundle connects to many parts of the brain that coordinate emotions. Stimulating this area of the brain was found to elicit both laughter and the emotions that come with it.[4]

What we find funny comes from our social, cultural and familial life experiences. As Norman Cousins affirmed: 'One man's humour is another man's ho-hum.'[5] I *know* my 'mum' jokes are hilarious; my family simply begs to differ. Although humour is not an emotion, it can affect our emotions. Even though not all humour or play results in laughter, it primes the mind's internal landscape for optimism and positivity. Different neurotransmitters are signalled, almost like a partition popping up in the brain – negative thoughts to one side, positive thoughts to the other.

Positive humour is generally associated with higher self-esteem, optimism and life satisfaction, with a reduction in depression, anxiety and stress. It is a means of expressing our humanity in an empathetic and kind way. As Robin Williams put it, 'With comedy you are allowed to laugh about the insanity, you realise how absurd it all is, the painful stuff and the wonderful stuff too. For a brief moment everyone is connected, and you all go "Hey, we're human".' On the other hand, negative humour (sarcasm, insults) can be damaging to mental health, resulting in sadness, not joy.

The multifaceted personality of humour can be understood through the Humor Styles Questionnaire, which classifies four uses of individual humour. Two are positively related to psychosocial health and wellbeing; the others are negative. These humour styles may be self-enhancing, affiliative (enhance one's relationships with others), aggressive (enhance the self at the expense of others) or self-defeating (enhance relationships at the expense of self). Males scored higher than females on aggressive and self-defeating humour.[6] Brain-imaging studies also suggest that men and women perceive humour differently.

The arts is one of the few areas where negative humour styles enjoy the limelight. Think Shakespeare's comedic insults, such as, 'Thou art as fat as butter' from *Henry IV*, or in more modern times satirical theatre, films and TV shows that relish the darker side of comedy: *Book of Mormon*, *Little Shop of Horrors*, *Avenue Q*, *The Producers*, *Jojo Rabbit*, *Death at a Funeral*, *South Park*, *Rick and Morty*, *Black Books* and Monty Python, replete with limbs lopped off and blood gushing everywhere, or a giant foot mercilessly squashing its underling. Where your humour barometer lies is in how much playing with darkness tickles your fancy. There's a fine line between satire and farce, tragedy and comedy.

. . . .

Like mittens mould to the shape of our hands, so too does our humour-print – which develops a little later than our laugh-print, from as early as seven months. Our sense of humour serves us over our lifespan, satiating an important social function more than a response to anything particularly funny. Humour is a vital accompaniment for children as they learn new things and respond to the environment around them. With a highly adaptive sense, what stimulates amusement or laughter in children visibly changes as quickly as their shoe size. From peek-a-boo hysterics to funny animal sounds, then onto a phase many parents fear may never end – toilet humour.

Like all kids, my son relished fart humour. One memory is etched in my mind: an interview with the principal of my son's soon-to-be primary school.

'What are you looking forward to about coming to the big school?' the kindly principal asked.

'Poo, poo, poo,' my son responded. Mortified, I nudged said child of mine to consider a more thoughtful response, to which he looked up and repeated matter-of-factly, 'Poo, poo, poo.'

Thankfully, the interview was more a formality than an evaluation, and within a few weeks, he joined the school's ranks, in his oversized uniform, blissfully unaware he had sullied our illustrious (ha, ha, ha) family name.

Our humour sense is so highly attuned to human development that, like children, it passes through adolescence. Anything remotely inappropriate, such as a teacher's bad hair day or mixing one's words while delivering a presentation, is hilarious. Then there is S. E. X. If only sex was as funny in real life as it is in adolescent minds! During this phase, when pimples and body parts are seemingly popping out of nowhere, humour is often drawn on to disguise angst. Although, it can become a little snarky when teenagers are competing for a place in the social hierarchy.

Like cheese, our sense of humour matures, informed by our life experiences – good and bad. What we found funny as children may no longer tickle our funny bone the more sophisticated it becomes and attuned to life's stresses. We find humour in situations as a way of trying to make sense of difficult matters. It strengthens our immunity to stress, among other things. Spiders, for one! One study showed humour therapy was just as effective as traditional desensitisation for arachnophobia.[7]

It's possible that our immunity improves because regularly activating our humour-side keeps us strong. It is, after all, a strength and is listed in the Values-in-Action (VIA) classification of twenty-four strengths and six universal virtues.[8] Humour was found to be compatible with all virtues, most strongly with humanity, wisdom and transcendence.[9] Impacting body, mind and spirit, humour is found in the transcendence category (no surprise) along with appreciation of beauty and excellence, gratitude, hope and spirituality. People with humour as one of their top character traits, also known as signature strengths, tend to concentrate on positive aspects of their past, present and future. Perhaps best summed up by this joke:

The past, present and future walk into a bar.
It was tense.

Existing purely in our mind and not the physical world, humour defies rules of convention. Sparkles of humour and laughter can be found in the least likely of places, during the darkest of times. Austrian neurologist, psychiatrist and author of *Man's Search for Meaning*, Viktor Frankl moved between four concentration camps over three years, including Auschwitz, where his brother died and his mother was killed. While imprisoned, Frankl wisely didn't leave humour to chance. Together with a friend, he made a promise to invent at least one amusing story daily about some incident that could happen one day after liberation. While he may have been starving, his imagination was fed. Humour enabled a practice of the art of living and momentary levity despite being in concentration camps and suffering being omnipresent. Even though his stories were future-orientated, they influenced the present moment – elevating him beyond the painful present to a more hopeful future. Humour enabled people to still feel like human beings – the one thing the Nazis did their darndest to destroy. It helped people rise above everyday existence to a different realm, where the same rules didn't apply. A form of 'spiritual resistance', jokes were used as weapons; humour and laughter were a power. Hitler himself was concerned about this, bemoaning in one of his speeches as to why Jews laughed at him. The Führer may have felt invincible on the battlefield as his tanks rolled over Europe, but one of his greatest fears was being laughed at.[10]

It could almost be argued that humour was made for adversity. Holocaust survivors recounted how a person with a healthy sense of humour was able to bear more.[11] Humour contributed to emotional survival, whether it was expressed as caricatures, satirical songs or theatrical performances. Comedians and jesters spread some lightness amid the fear and overcrowding that existed in the Warsaw and Łódź ghettos. 'Humour is not for the long term, it is for the moment,' shared one survivor. As long as there was laughter there was hope. While there was laughter, there was life. Amid hopelessness, the odd chuckle, witticism and occasional joke was shared. Even if for only a short while, it allowed people to retreat to 'a world that has been made whole and in which the miseries of the human condition have been abolished'.[12] As author Mark Twain penned,

'The human race has one really effective weapon, and that is laughter.'

Tuning into humour when life's a bed of roses is easy. The challenge is seizing humorous moments when it's a bed of thorns. That's where the Laughter Effect comes in. I commandeered this philosophy years ago, when checking in at the hospital counter to have my bowel reconnected. 'I'm checking in with two bags, but will be leaving with one,' I joked with the nurse. It took a moment for the penny to drop, for her to realise that I was referring to relinquishing my ileostomy bag. This was my way of defusing nervous energy and fear, of which I had plenty. It had been a tough few months. Understatement. My sense of humour verged on a non-sense, which is why I needed to dig deep. I joked with hospital staff about my reason for the timing of my operation – bananas! A whopping cyclone had obliterated Australia's banana supply and prices were exorbitant, if you could source them at all. But the hospital kitchen supplied me with as many bananas as I liked. Finding the funniness of it made me feel better, and sharing jocularity also brightened the spirits of attending nurses. They'd leave the room smiling, increasing the probability of the Laughter Effect travelling to the next patient.

Going through two major operations within a few months was tough on my whole family, especially my boys. Mindful of this, I endeavoured to make light of my situation. After my bowel was reconnected, I was advised the first sign of business as usual would be if I could fart. Leading up to this momentous event, my son Zak would call the hospital daily and enquire as to whether I'd farted. On day three, post-op, I could barely reach for my phone quick enough to share my exciting news. I relished the echoes of delight as Zak relayed my news on the other end of the phone to the rest of the family, 'Mum's farted, Mum's farted!' It just goes to show, fart humour is effective at all ages. My humour response fed into the family's humour response, allowing a much-needed dose of laughter to break the cycle of fear and tension. At times, life is too serious to be taken seriously! As author and 'jollytologist' Allen Klein says in *The Healing Power of Humor*, 'sometimes we do not see the importance of laughter in our dark times because we are so blinded by our tears'. He further asserts 'the pain may not stop but humour can reduce suffering and give someone a sense of agency and control despite the overall helpless situation'.

Humour psychologist Steve Sultanoff provides the perspective that 'humour helps us experience happiness. And when we experience happiness, other emotions disappear such as depression, anxiety and anger – at least for a little while – since it is impossible to experience happiness, anger and fear simultaneously'. Negative emotions are often stored deep within, rather than expressed. Laughter and humour provide a way for these emotions to be harmlessly released.

Fear is our body's equivalent to quicksand. It is immobilising and constrictive. Cultivating levity encourages a more expansive mindset. It helps broaden and build positive emotions, as suggested by Professor of Positive Psychology Barbara Fredrickson in the Broaden-and-Build theory. It's based on the notion of the ripple effect of positive emotions, broadening awareness and response to events, as well as building personal resources and coping skills that can enhance resilience to stress in the future.[13] When we can laugh at our pain, or gain a fresh perspective on it, some of the associated trauma melts away. This enables our brain to recall a challenging time or life event with less sting. And so 'The Day of the Fart' is recalled, bringing a smile to the memory of that time, instead of focusing on the physical pain or fear that my bowel may never again function properly.

In this, I assumed a lead role in initiating humour. Coming from staff, the joke would have been a calculated risk, which is why humour's use in a therapeutic context is often underplayed. Yet research conducted in the Netherlands with medical oncologists in a comprehensive cancer centre found humour helped relieve stress associated with disease and illness. Humour was reportedly used by 97 per cent of oncology specialists. They all reported laughing at times during consultations and 83 per cent experienced a positive effect of laughter.[14]

You might be thinking, *A Dutch study, no wonder they were laughing,* but I can assure you that no green leafy props were used. Despite medical complications, patients found humour beneficial in broaching difficult topics and downplaying challenges. It wasn't always successful, though. Sometimes humour was viewed as inappropriate – largely because of a difference in taste. However, it helped to ease emotional pain by demonstrating the human side of the healthcare team. It allowed everyone to cope and build positive relationships, especially when it was a conscious choice of the patient.[15] As it had been mine.

Gallows humour (making fun of life-threatening or other serious situations) should be avoided. And one of the most damaging and dismissive things you can do is to tell someone to laugh off their woes. It's essential to take the cue from the individual patient. Are they ready to laugh about or at their pain? As comedian Steve Martin quipped, 'First the doctor told me the good news: I was going to have a disease named after me.'

A MOMENT OF LEVITY IN GRAVITY

Can you recall a time when humour (resulting in laughter) alleviated a stressful situation?
Did you initiate it or did someone else?
How did a laughter response impact your stress levels at the time?
As you recall this scenario now, what aspect of it do you connect to the most? The stressful side or the unanticipated funny one?

When it comes to a sense of humour, use common sense

Humour's beauty is in the eye of the beholder. In a crisis or serious situation, whether a type of humour is viewed negatively or positively depends on what meaning you place on the particular crisis and how it impacted you emotionally. Let's cast our mind back to the early days of Covid, when the lack of toilet paper supply was a bit of a joke. However, if you joke about Covid with someone who lost a loved one to it, you're playing with fire. There is a vast difference between the humour in the decimation of toilet paper supply and the actual decimation of lives. Generally, Tragedy + X Time = Humour. But in this case, no passage of time might be enough. The X is the stickiness component – how emotionally 'sticky' the event still feels. As Steve Sultanoff explains: 'Individuals with some distance from the crisis are less likely to experience a merging of self and the crisis. Those with some distance may be aided by humour because it reinforces perspective and creates a safe distance from the crisis.'[16]

Yet a fear of being insensitive or not taking critical life events seriously means people often refrain from sharing humour or applying it to their own circumstances. It can be considered taboo, where guilt is associated with expressing positive emotions in the face of adversity; humour is absent when needed the most.

One of my clients had lost both her parents over a twelve-month period. Devastated, she deprived herself of feeling joy for more than a year, believing anything other than grief would disrespect their memory. She was numb and no longer laughing or smiling with her partner. We pieced together a plan. Her first step was to grant herself permission to feel positive emotions again. She needed to accept that her parents would not want her to be trampled by grief. I then encouraged her to verbalise and journal times when they had all laughed together. Shedding some tears along the way, we practised smiling and laughing, welcoming joy back into her life. My client went on to view comedies with her partner, and slowly but surely laughter came back into their relationship. Within weeks, her mood lifted, as did the intimate relationship both with herself and her partner. Laughter allowed a break from the heaviness of reality.

Naturally, a degree of sensitivity and common sense is needed when sharing or inviting humour with individuals in the wake of pain, trauma

CASE STUDY: Dumb Ways to Die

We've grown accustomed to fear tactics scaring us into changing unhealthy behaviours. The Grim Reaper AIDS campaign from the 1980s still sends shockwaves down my spine. However, there's another proven way to capture our attention and influence behaviour – humour. Mingling facts with funny has resulted in some of the most impactful public health social marketing campaigns. In Australia, messaging on poor safety behaviour around trains had largely fallen on deaf ears. That was until Metro Trains changed tracks, adopting the marketing campaign devised by advertising agency McCann, 'Dumb Ways to Die'. The song and video's main messaging, 'poor safety around trains means you are dumb', struck a chord.

Dumb Ways to Die drew on offbeat humour, an incredibly catchy tune and a cast of endearing animated characters. Think SpongeBob SquarePants with a touch of Minions. Appealing to all ages, the humour in it underscored the many dumb ways to die: 'Set fire to your hair, poke a stick at a grizzly bear, eat medicine that's out of date, use your private parts as piranha bait ... sell both your kidneys on the internet, eat a tube of superglue, take your helmet off in outer space ...', before concluding with the campaign's primary message: 'stand on the edge of a train station platform, drive around the boom gates at a level crossing, run across the tracks between the platforms, they may not rhyme but they're quite possibly the dumbest ways to die'.

The video went viral, viewed 2.5 million times within forty-eight hours and 4.7 million times within seventy-two hours, and has now amassed over 300 million views. The 'Dumb Ways to Die' song was in the iTunes top 10 chart, and the Google Play Games app had nearly 4 billion (not a typo) mini-game plays within three months of its launch, making the song a record-breaker for the most shared ad. Most importantly, following the campaign Metro Trains found a 21 per cent reduction in train-station accidents and deaths and, to date, more than 127 million people have pledged they will be safer around trains because of the campaign. More than dumb luck, its brand of humour changed lives.

or grief. The two-faced nature of humour calls for constant assessment and reflection to ensure its appropriate and timely use. If you need to explain or justify its use, then the humour has likely backfired. As the late Clive James – critic, journalist, author and broadcaster – wrote: 'Common sense and a sense of humour are the same thing, moving at different speeds. A sense of humour is just common sense dancing.'

The Laughter Effect not only elevates humour at an individual level, but it can also have a profound collective impact. In fact, it can even change the course of history! At an Association of Applied Therapeutic Humor (AATH) conference, where humour is taken very seriously, comedian and guest speaker Yakov Smirnoff regaled tales of humour's peace-making ability. Originally from Soviet Russia, he and his family were taken in by the United States in 1977, when he was twenty-six. Humour became his lifeline, helping him navigate the culture gap between the East and West. He even adopted a more 'user-friendly' surname – Smirnoff – inspired by his first job in his new home country as a bartender in the Catskills, where comedians would frequent.

It wasn't long before his star began to shine. One day his phone rang. On the other end of the line, a male voice. Someone purporting to be President Reagan. It took Smirnoff a little while to realise this was no stunt. Reagan loved Smirnoff's jokes and considered him a master of one-liners. He believed Smirnoff to be the perfect comedian to lighten his Cold War speech, which he planned on delivering at the Kremlin at the Moscow Summit in 1988. The political landscape between the United States and Russia was tense. The humour stakes were high. Reagan opened his addressed with Smirnoff's joke, one that strongly implied that heaven itself had endowed communist politicians with lazy asses. It was a gamble. Watching on his TV in his lounge room at home in the United States, Smirnoff was terrified. And it looked like his fears were coming to fruition in a room full of Communist Party apparatchiks, stony-faced, most of all Gorbachev. Smirnoff's stomach dropped to the floor. He was a *goner*. But then a moment later, the room broke into applause. He hadn't factored in the delay for the translation to kick in. The ice had been broken. The talks resumed and the rest is history.

Whether it's an issue of global consequence or a more personal one, the disarming and distracting nature of humour helps deflect from the issue at hand. While in residential care, my dad suffered a nasty fall and was rushed to hospital in an ambulance. Dad looked like he had fallen prey to a warring blackberry bush. Yet he was remarkably alert and in good cheer. Perhaps the knock on his head had somehow reawakened his Alzheimer's-riddled mind, like a scene from *Patch Adams,* whom he now resembled, with a mismatch of gauze pads and dressings and, on my insistence, a smattering of smiley-faced plasters usually reserved for children. The smiley faces distracted me from his puffed-up, bruised face, while simultaneously generating lovely compliments and courteous laughter from attending staff. Despite still being in Emergency, it was a relief to enjoy some micro-moments of lightheartedness.

Humour in the workplace

By the time people enter the workforce, there's a tendency to fall off a 'humour cliff' – both in laugh frequency and self-perception of funniness. According to Jennifer Aaker and Naomi Bagdonas, who teach the popular course Humor: Serious Business at the Stanford Graduate School of Business, there's a belief that frivolity won't serve us well in our professional lives. As such, our laughter- and humour-selves go into recession – a Global Humour Cliff (GHC), a personal equivalent to the Global Financial Crisis (GFC). This has been demonstrated in a Gallup poll that asked people in 166 countries the simple question, 'Did you smile or laugh yesterday?' In the sixteen-to-twenty age group, the answer was largely 'yes'. By age twenty-three, the response was largely 'no'. It wasn't until the senior years, aged seventy and over, that the response returned to 'yes'. Gratefully, some of us reach this realisation ahead of others.

The average person spends one-third of their life at work. That's around 90,000 hours over the course of a lifetime. I'm not sure who Ms or Mr Average is, but that's a huge chunk of time to precariously hang off a cliff. Move over traditional MBAs, hello Mirth Blissful Amusement. Punchlines can enhance bottom lines, improving work satisfaction, performance, health and team cohesion.

According to a workplace-based survey, 91 per cent of executives believe a sense of humour is important for career advancement and 84 per cent feel that people with a good sense of humour do a better job.[17] Bell Leadership Institute found a sense of humour was one of the two most desirable traits in leaders, the other being a strong work ethic.[18] Note, humour inspired by the smash hit *The Office* – where leaders try to be funny and fail, engage in negative humour styles like sarcasm, or make fun of themselves or others – runs the risk of backfiring rather than firing up.

Using appropriate positive humour is an acquired skill that improves with practice. Understanding what hits the humour mark in your workplace can take time but, when you do, it is ever so rewarding. Rather than distract from important duties, humour helps you get things done, motivating others by dissolving tension and calming conflict. Humour is a cheerleader for your team, peers and colleagues. Leaders engaging their humerus are viewed as more motivating and admired. According to Jennifer Aaker, employees are 15 per cent more engaged and satisfied in their jobs, and rate their leaders as 27 per cent more motivating.[19]

Humour helps shift cognitive energy from the limbic or emotional system to our wiser prefrontal cortex. This means sharper thinking, better problem-solving, increased creativity and improved ability to forecast the future. Humour's ability to create a bond and build trust helps decrease arrogance, with people more likely to be receptive to feedback (an important attribute in any workplace). As former US president Eisenhower said, 'A sense of humour is part of the art of leadership, of getting along with people, of getting things done.'

If being funny is not your strong point, don't fret. Delegate someone in your workplace to take the lead. A humour ambassador responsible for gainful giggles, if you like. Doing so is a smart move, according to neurohumorist Karyn Buxman: 'Humour is a vital tool in regaining and maintaining our ability to think clearly. When we're stressed, our IQ drops more than ten points.' That's because your brain is too busy putting out the fires to solve problems creatively, if at all. Buxman calls this the 'cognitive capacity cascade'.

Hilarity may be the solution, saving your company thousands of dollars on organisational psychology. Teams that laugh together before trying to solve a creativity challenge are more than twice as likely to succeed versus those who don't. But there's more. Adding a jovial line like 'And my final offer is X amount of dollars and I'll throw in my pet frog' at the end of a sales pitch created an 18 percent leap in customers' willingness to pay more.[20]

Humour pays off – literally. Rather than being frowned upon, positive humour in the workplace is a key to better performance. Just think how many lives you will save from falling off the precipice too.

. . . .

Humour not only helps solve problems, but it can also help solve crimes. In a study of crime investigators, humour and joking played an important role in reducing stress and facilitating teamwork in a high-pressure environment. Humour served to reduce stress so that job tasks could be completed. It was also used as a barometer of the investigators' negotiation of the emotional burdens of such work.[21] One assumes gallows humour was their preferred method of humour execution.

SEROTONIN SISTER

I'm not particularly funny. How can I develop my sense of humour?

Be on the lookout for things that ignite your humour and share them with colleagues, friends and loved ones – whether you do that on social media, by recounting something funny you heard or memorising a joke you can drop into conversations. This will train your brain to scan for humorous happenings and grow your humour capacity. The more positive feedback you receive, the more your confidence will grow.

HUMOUR JOURNAL

Collect and share things that make you laugh and add humour
to your life to relieve stress – quotes, memes or funny photos.
Compile these in a journal. On days you're feeling a little flat, spend
time flicking through your journal, or search for something fun
or funny to add. Hanging out in the lighter side of life will tilt your
smile upward and buoy your spirit.

The belly laugh battle of the sexes

Due to humour's subjective nature, sensitivity needs to be considered
when it comes to individual humour styles and cultural and gender
differences. It's a rule that applies wherever you are in the globe, even
in space!

Spending weeks or even months in space can be a lonely business.
Astronauts endure many internal and external stressors – although
what to wear each day is not one of them. One study found astronauts
using positive humour demonstrated lower levels of loneliness, depression, stress, tension and anxiety, and an improvement in their overall
wellbeing. Humour also increased feelings of togetherness, warmth,
friendliness and led to high levels of self-esteem and optimism. Important for anyone, but especially when you're cooped up with the same
person day-in, day-out for a lengthy period. Using humour to cope
was also reported to improve empathy among crew and helped communication. [22]

Consistent with other research on gender differences in humour,
female astronauts were less likely to use humour as a coping strategy.
In general, males are more likely to use humour, especially at work.[23]
Humour as a coping mechanism was used more in experienced cosmo-
nauts, whereas greenhorns were more prone to go into problem-solving

mode. Women were found to use a greater degree of executive processing and language-based decoding when processing humour.[24] Proving the point that men are from Mars and women are from Venus. In summary, gravity mixed with gravity = LEVITY.

Defying gravity

Defying gravity helps us age well. At any age and stage of life, humour is important, especially as we enter our twilight years. It's a vital coping mechanism to help diminish the impact of life's transformations, illness and loss – of independence and loved ones. One of the top regrets of many people towards the end of their life is not having laughed more. Finding the humour in everyday situations is nature's antioxidant. A regular dose of HRT (Humour Replacement Therapy) keeps our hormones happy. As Jennifer Aaker says, 'It's like exercising, meditating and having sex all at the same time!'

Sparking the Laughter Effect through humour is a protective, natural and empowering response. Our sixth sense invites levity, making us more resilient and confident to tackle whatever may come next. Like any skill, it needs to be consciously practised until it becomes innate. If you have stopped seeing the funny in the small things that go awry, there's less chance you'll be able to see it in the larger things. And a word of caution: please do whatever it takes to prevent falling off the humour cliff. As American writer, publisher, artist and philosopher Elbert Hubbard said, 'Do not take life too seriously. You'll never get out of it alive.'

HUMOUR HABITS

What humour habits can you introduce in your life, both personally and professionally? Be specific about what is required, who is involved and your desired outcome.

Some ideas:

→ Ahead of a birthday party, organise for people to write down funny memories about the birthday guest. Read these out. You'll be amazed that even if people recall the same event, how they express and remember this event will differ.

→ Create funny acronyms to describe a project you're working on.

→ Brush up on your jokes.

→ Write captions for cartoons and come up with jokes in response to everyday frustrating situations.

→ Share your favourite tongue-twister, at home or at work.

6

Playing with the Laughter Effect

Your body cannot heal without play. Your mind cannot heal without laughter. Your soul cannot heal without joy
— Catherine Rippenger Fenwick

Child's play

We've seen how humour and laughter are integral to the Laughter Effect – so too is play. We are born to play. Even if it doesn't result in laugh-out-loud moments, play puts the body and mind in a positive emotional state. Whether structured or organic, play opens our minds, promoting imagination and creativity. Important at any stage of life, it's a social, cognitive and emotional strength, facilitating the development of skills and resources. Its universal ability to forge social bonds lends itself to being a strength of humanity.

Sadly, play is too often restricted to the playground and left behind in our childhood. Yet evolutionarily we're wired to play. In Darwin's observations of apes playing, he noted playful panting sounds shared the same acoustic structure as human laughter, prompting a necessary tweak to this happy birthday parody from 'you look like a monkey, and you smell like one too' to 'you look like a monkey, and you laugh like one too'. In *The Expression of the Emotions in Man and Animals*, he highlighted laughter, a natural response to play, as a primary expression of joy.

Children's constant laughter while playing sends reassurance to adults that all is well, that there's no need to intervene. Child's play blends physical, mental and make-believe elements. It is critical for development of a baby's nervous system and brain networks. Smiling is often the first sign of an invitation to play, whereas laughter generally happens during interactive play. Playfulness in a group is the social setting for most laughs. The more play, the more laughter: the more laughter, the more play!

Children who laugh together, grow together, with mutual laughter assisting synchronised learning. Play is a stimulant for humour development – a novel way to express oneself. As Albert Einstein said: 'Having fun is the best way to learn.' Some examples of playful learning include scientific experiments where children create soda bombs with Coke and Mentos mints; or playing with bubbles, slime and playdough. Play is fundamental to becoming a fully-fledged social being.

It can take a crisis to bring on play. During the peak of the Covid-19 pandemic, TikTok was bursting with quarantined parents, even grandparents, transforming kitchens into sound studios, and even mastering Irish dancing. Being playful and having fun, especially in households, sent a clear signal that while the external world was far from perfect at the time, there was freedom in choosing how to respond. Playing outside the hopscotch square revealed a fresh perspective to a challenging situation. Parents dancing around the living room, having fun and being silly conveyed a sense of ease and paved the way for positive emotions to emerge, such as joy, love and gratitude. Drawing on humour, play teaches both big kids and little kids that there's another way to respond to conflict and crisis. Playing to distract or reframe helps to develop personal resilience.

Kids are natural players. Over a lifetime, play becomes more intellectual and less spontaneous. As part of my research for this book, I wanted to take a pulse from the playground. Was there a connection between adults laughing less than children because they play less? I posed a question to a group of children: 'Who plays more, kids or adults?' They sized me up, certain I was joking with them. Surely it was obvious. 'Adults have to work, so they can't play,' they snickered. Adults don't work all the time, I countered, so could there be another reason? A little voice chimed, 'Kids are funner!' That put the matter fairly and squarely to rest, for the moment.

COLLECTING CHILDHOOD HAPPY MEMORIES

Time travel back to your childhood. Make a list of all the things that brought you joy when you were young. Allow yourself to daydream and relive these memories as if they were happening today. During this process of recollecting happy memories, is there anywhere in your body you notice these sensations the most? If there is, expand and deepen this feeling. Breathe into it, smile into it, acknowledge the joy.

Joking around

While kids might be *funner*, their ability to tell jokes comes with age, as joke-telling is a more mature evolution than instinctual laughter. I am clearly under-evolved, suffering from joke amnesia – frequently forgetting the punchline or garbling it in the set-up. Others are born jokers. Freud frequently used jokes in his analytical work with his patients. He asserted, 'A new joke is passed around from one person to another like the news of the latest victory.'[1] This observation couldn't be truer as we witnessed a virtual *pundemic* alongside the pandemic, with humorous memes flooding social media while sorry statistics dominated mainstream press. The Freudism that 'a joke is truth wrapped in a smile' serves two purposes: aggression, such as sarcasm; or to expose unconscious desires via sexual jokes. Freud theorised that the more repressed sexual feeling a person has, the more they will enjoy sexual jokes, releasing mental energy, allowing access to one's unconscious mind.[2] In other words, jokes are an opportunity to derive enjoyment from something one cannot usually enjoy any other way. He richly observed the physical response of laughing at a joke as 'leading our diaphragm to pulsate and chest to heave, releasing psychic energy that would otherwise have been used to repress our anxiety about death that the joke expresses!'[3]

Freud noted how jokes rely on an exchange between the teller and the recipient. A shared sense of playful camaraderie is achieved when joker and jokee laugh audibly, signalling they both 'get' it. In *The Joke and Its Relation to the Unconscious*, Freud further observed that 'a joke begins in play, deriving pleasure from the liberation of nonsense; but then it can rise to the help of major purposes such as combating suppression and fighting against the forces of critical judgement and oppression'.[4]

I'm not sure his deep insights apply to common or garden jokes such as:

What do Alexander the Great and Winnie the Pooh have in common?
The same middle name.

Most playful interactions and spur-of-the-moment jokes arise from responding to everyday experiences: mishaps, slips of the tongue, incongruities, social observations or puns. Yet sometimes, despite being imparted in jest, a joke cuts too close to the bone. It is these jokes Freud believed revealed the potential to discover something new or important about ourselves. Decades later, he continues to inspire a new generation of admirers, and jokes. Speaking of which:

What is a Freudian slip?
When you say one thing, but you mean your mother.

Jokes draw on elements of truth mixed with incongruity or misdirection. You're heading one way, but then go somewhere else. Point in case, by comedian Sarah Silverman: 'Once I was with two men in one night. But I could never do it again. I could hardly walk afterwards. Two dinners? That's a lot of food.'

My mother-in-law, Lillian, was a natural joke-teller. It was how her brain was wired. For years she was our personalised 'Old Jews Telling Jokes' streaming service. A natural extension of her free-flowing, unfiltered mind. She'd enquire, 'Have I told you this one, Ros?' to which I'd respond, 'Yes, many times.' This never dissuaded her from telling it again, and again, and again. One of her oft-told gems:

There's a retired couple, Betty and Abe. They're both becoming more forgetful. They're watching a Golden Oldie on TV when an ad comes on.

Betty says, 'Abe, I'm going to get some ice cream with strawberry topping. Would you like some?'

'Sure,' he says, 'but make sure you write it down or you might forget.'

'I'll remember,' she hastily remarks.

Quite a bit of time lapses.

Abe shouts out to the other end of the house, 'Betty, what's taking you so long? The film has started again.'

Finally, he hears her footsteps getting louder down the corridor and he relaxes back into his seat.

She hands him a plate of scrambled eggs.

He takes one look at the eggs and exclaims, 'You see, I told you you'd forget something. Where's my toast?'

Lillian's playful joke-telling was an endearing characteristic. Let's just say it helped soothe the inevitable frustrations of family dynamics (in my other life I am a diplomat). It was a charm that drew strangers to her like a magnet. Her joke-telling repertoire ensured her inner child remained intact.

Opening ourselves up to play

Play is a state of mind. We hold the baton. Without a playful attitude, an event might be interpreted in many ways – scary, puzzling, silly or frustrating, but certainly not funny. Haven't we all experienced this, when we're not in the mood for frivolity and nothing will rouse our fun-loving self? The absence of a playful mind disables the processing of humorous stimuli.

Play has liberating characteristics, relaxing the need for control and opening the mind to new possibilities. Author Mark Matousek notes in *Writing to Awaken: A Journey of Truth, Transformation and Self-Discovery*, 'To be serious on our path to awakening means that we learn how to play.' In doing so, we connect to our wiser, more passionate and creative side, to a fresh perspective that encourages our brains to discover new possibilities. Or as David Cronin, Australian clown doctor, laughter yogi and author of *Breathe Play Laugh*, commented, 'It's like all the lights in your house are on and you have access to every room.'

Jocularity lights up our brain – almost literally. Research using an electroencephalogram (EEG) was used to examine brain activity when participants viewed humorous material and it identified Joke Central – the areas of the brain that light up in response to a humour stimulus.[5] Within 4/10ths of a second, researchers observed an electrical wave moving to the cerebral cortex in the left hemisphere of the brain, where words and the structure of jokes are analysed, and the right hemisphere, where intellectual processing takes place. Social emotional responses take place in the frontal lobe, and visual signals (smiling) and motor responses (laughter) in the occipital lobe. It appears that the right hemisphere of our brain has the last laugh. If it becomes impaired through injury or disease, so too can a person's ability to process humour, laughter or even a smile.[6]

Pioneer in the humour field, Dr Paul McGhee has devised a Sense of Humour scale in which play is critical. McGhee identifies eight areas of humour-related behaviours: (1) enjoyment of humour, (2) seriousness/negative mood, (3) playfulness/positive mood, (4) laughter, (5) verbal humour, (6) finding humour in everyday life, (7) laughing at yourself and (8) humour under stress. Note this last one is the most difficult to develop.[7] A rating system generates a Humour Quotient: the higher, the better. McGhee believes 'your sense of humour is a form of play – mental play or play with ideas'.

Play can be expressed in many ways – wordplay, board games, online games, jokes, witty banter, physical play, the list goes on. In some people, a sense of play rules while in others it's an undertone. There's a vulnerability associated with playfulness, where the untamed version of our raw self is laid bare. Being seen to be silly can be interpreted by some as a source of shame. Vulnerability is such a universal quality that we often don't recognise it's there until something brings it to our attention. American psychiatrist, clinical researcher and founder of the US National Institute on Play, Dr Stuart Brown acknowledges laughing hysterically can make us feel a little out of control. Revealing our playful side can position us outside our comfort zone.

Avoiding awkwardness and judgement is one of many explanations why our playful side becomes shy. *What will people think? Grow up! You look ridiculous, get a handle on yourself.* Or as my parents spatted, 'Rosalind, settle down.' It's only by embracing our playful self that we have more confidence in engaging in play. Otherwise, it may remain in hiding – trapped in a never-ending game of hide and seek.

Endowed with insight, Eleanor Roosevelt proclaimed, 'You don't grow up until you have your first good laugh at yourself.' Humans are

Of the many flights I've taken over the years, one stands out. Not because of pockets of turbulence or fidgety kids kicking the back of my seat, but because of the jokes. Southwest Airlines do things a little differently. Rather than rows of serious or anxious faces on passengers, you're more likely to hear and see smiles and laughter. Its organisational culture has put the fun back into flying, not only for passengers but also for employees. Part of the company pledge is to 'Express my Fun-LUVing Attitude by not taking myself too seriously'. And in their slate of values under the banner of humility: 'Don't take yourself too seriously; keep perspective', and my favourite, 'Don't be a jerk.'

With around 40 per cent of the population experiencing some form of anxiety about flying, of these 2.5 to 5 per cent facing crippling anxiety, incorporating frivolity and laughter as part of the in-flight service makes sense. For Southwest, punchlines have also made good business sense, with an independent consulting group finding that telling jokes during the safety demonstrations resulted in US$140 million of revenue per year.[8] This joke, for example, relayed seven times per week amounts to a cool $0.0000002 million each time it's told: 'Put the oxygen mask on yourself first, then on your child. If you're travelling with more than one child, start with the one who has more potential or who is less likely to put you in a home.'

While not all humour tickles everyone's fancy, proximity of passengers to one another promotes the likelihood of contagious laughter and at a minimum elevates the vibe. Jocularity underpins the flight service, from the captain's welcome onboard message: 'Ladies and gentlemen, welcome aboard this Southwest flight to Denver. We will be taking off just as soon as I can get through page ten of this flight manual', to flight attendants appealing to scrambling passengers to place bags in the overhead luggage compartments, jesting, 'If your cabin luggage doesn't fit in the overhead bins, we'll be happy to put it on eBay for you.'

Even at the journey's end, one particular baggage handler has been known to harmonise a moment by whipping out his ukulele, remarking, 'No one can frown when you're listening to a ukulele.'

It's not just about jokes, Southwest is also the perfect embodiment of the Laughter Effect, and I say that not because I'd love to be compensated with free flights. While most airlines were reeling from the pandemic and fastening their fiscal seatbelts, in 2021 Southwest Airlines celebrated their fiftieth year by inspiring 1 million Acts of Kindness, donating Southwest travel awards to fifty-two organisations that championed kindness throughout their communities.

Their holistic approach extends to commendation of staff in company newsletters, CEO messages of praise streamed in staff meetings, and dinners where meals are served on a retractable tray (not really) honouring a noteworthy employee. Compliments received on social media or other means of communication are forwarded to both employee and their manager. On average over 7000 compliments a month are received – especially impressive as most airlines are dogged by an ever-increasing number of complaints.[9] No wonder voluntary turnover at Southwest sits at 2 per cent and it's rated number one for the lowest number of customer complaints. If your attitude determines your altitude, Southwest is soaring high. In my opinion, the only thing missing is a Smile High Club!

not machines and need to be motivated, whether they're infants or adults. Despite popular belief, appropriate humour at work can be a way to safely express our vulnerabilities. Regrettably, in today's culture, self-worth is often tied to our productivity, meaning spending time on play seems counterproductive. Decades before the iPhone, in the early 1900s, philosopher Bertrand Russell wrote in *In Praise of Idleness* that 'there was formerly a capacity for lightheartedness and play, which has to some extent been inhibited by the cult of efficiency'. Seems we have a bit of a way to catch up with the past.

From workplace to work play

Dr Stuart Brown highlights the purposelessness of play as to why many companies view it as a waste of time. However, it's not like a corporation needs to commit to completing a game of Monopoly until all houses are bought and someone's in the clanger; it's the small playful interactions that set the tone. These are what motivate us to continue the task at hand, especially when obstacles come our way, helping us attain a goal, small or large, with the associated dopamine rush. Playful interactions give our rational mind time out. The intentional use of playful humour also increases relational empathy, building trust. An Australian industry study of 2500 employees found 81 per cent believed a fun working environment would make them more productive, 93 per cent said that laughing on the job helps to reduce work-related stress, and 55 per cent said they would take less pay to have more fun at work.[10] Any CEOs or financial controllers may want to take note – but please don't interpret this as an excuse for docking pay.

In recent years, workplaces have gone to the dogs. By that I mean more companies have been encouraging employees to bring their pooches to the office. There's even an International Take Your Dog to Work Day in June! What better way to activate play, fun and joy than with a

SEROTONIN SISTER

I'm not naturally playful unless a serious game of Scrabble can be counted. Around children I feel less self-conscious. How can I become more playful without feeling silly?

Very few people relish the idea of being outside their comfort zone. Start slow and choose your audience. Kids can be less judgemental. As most adults feel less self-conscious expressing their playful side around kids, that's a good audience with which to start. Despite believing being silly is a 'bad' thing, it's actually healthy. In case you were wondering, silly and stupid are two different things, as a little bit of silly can free yourself of stress, resulting in greater creativity and improved mood. Keep in mind that play comes in many forms – physical, formal or even intellectual. Perhaps experiment with witty banter in the company of more mature folks who mightn't be as open to silliness?

four-legged friend? They help relieve stress and anxiety as their bonding and smelly breath weaves magic, reducing cortisol and stimulating oxytocin and other hormones associated with positive wellbeing. Dogs are a great excuse to legitimately be a little silly, connect to our inner child and also see the playful side of co-workers. A hard-nosed boss who encounters a wet nose and waggly tail may be transformed into a fun-loving human being, as opposed to an abrasive 'human doing'. Dogs in the workplace make us less vulnerable to vulnerability!

Time and again I witness vulnerability demons, especially during corporate Laughter Yoga sessions when there is no choice to opt out, nowhere to run, nowhere to hide. Sometimes I wonder whether people would be less resistant if I asked them to strip down to their underwear – a well-known vulnerability trigger. Another Dr Brown – Dr Brené Brown, legendary professor at the University of Houston – has conducted extensive research on courage, vulnerability, shame and empathy. She views laughter as a major component of shame resilience. Rather than connecting and fostering meaningful relationships, for many it disconnects, feeding into a sense of fear. Moving away from shame requires moving towards empathy, which takes compassion. Facing our vulnerabilities takes immense courage, but doing so opens the door to laughing and playing without fear of being judged or laughed at.

WORK PLAY

'Two truths and a lie' is a fun ice-breaker game, playfully blending humour with vulnerability. As part of a meeting or wellbeing day, ask each member of your team to reveal two truths and a lie about themselves. The rest of your team needs to guess which one is the lie.

According to psychologist Dr Michael Gervais, one of the greatest crip-plers of potential is Fear Of People's Opinions (FOPO). 'We play it safe and we play it small because we're afraid of what will happen on the other side of the critique,' Gervais contends.[11] There are few things worse than feeling embarrassed. Being laughed at feeds 'the sense of shame wolf', which is why sometimes a gentle reframe of laughter to joyful breath-work helps alleviate fear. Few would be condemned for how they breathe. In group Laughter Yoga sessions, once the silent nod of permission has been granted to let their hair down (bald people inclusive), there's a collective exhale. With sleeves rolled up and Windsor knots loosened, people relax into the play flow and the wall of shame and vulnerability comes tumbling down.

What you resist persists. If you don't honour your playful side, like a three-year-old, it will continue throwing a tantrum until it is allowed to play. From what I have witnessed over the years, there are a lot of three-year-olds dressed in suits! It's time for workplaces to become workplays.

Maximising learning through play

Author and co-founder of the Humour Academy at the Association for Applied and Therapeutic Humor, Mary Kay Morrison has come up with a dedicated name for these serious types – Humordoomers. As an educa-tor, Morrison has found that play and laughter maximise learning. Even the most reluctant learner will benefit from playing with the Laughter Effect, she maintains. A belief echoed by the professor of psychology at the University of Miami and author of *The Laughing Guide to* series, Isaac Prilleltensky, who explains how positive emotions engender creativity and problem-solving, so we literally become 'smarter through laughter', as the brain grows most rapidly when we are playing and having fun.

Morrison explains that motion drives attention, and attention drives learning – which explains why someone may not remember what you said but will remember how it made them feel. We also pay more attention if something takes us by surprise, which is what play and humour can do. At over seventy years of age, Morrison is the most fun person I know. Perhaps because she's a swinger. I should know, I've swung with her. Ha, not in that way! On a seat suspended by ropes. She has eleven swings on her property and seizes every opportunity to use them. Her personal mantra is, *Find time each day to play! If you're not sure what to do, think about what you loved to do as a child.*

Another adult who has resisted terminal seriousness is author and humorist Lenny Ravich, eighty-eight years young. For the bulk of his younger years, he suppressed his emotions. He wasn't aware he had any! Vulnerability and manhood went together like floral socks with open sandals at a formal soiree. A journey into Gestalt therapy altered Ravich's internal emotional landscape, exposing his vulnerabilities. With his emotions unleashed, he transformed his life. He identified four universal root emotions: mad, glad, sad and scared. In simply noticing where these emotions expressed themselves in his body, they began to calm down, he explained, 'like a kid tugging at your sleeve will stop as soon as you give them what they need'.

Ravich recounted the following example to me. One of the perks of being a senior is riding in the front of the bus. On one such trip in his hometown of Tel Aviv, Ravich boarded and hurriedly sat next to another senior who, Ravich swears, morphed into a snarling vampire, reprimanding Ravich for hitting him with his satchel. His reaction made Ravich feel mad! He could have yelled and screamed back, making a big scene, likely resulting in an active buy-in from other passengers (anyone who has spent any time in Israel will understand what I mean). He could have sweetly apologised, ignored him or thumped him again. Yet recognising the swell of anger in his chest, another – more playful – option came to mind. Ravich lifted his bag, stared at its leathery face and proceeded to whack it, saying, 'You naughty, naughty bag.' At first, he felt vulnerable – he wasn't sure how his approach would be met – but he instantly created intimacy. The snarling vampire became a smiling chum. Together they transitioned from mad to glad. Observing Ravich's twinkle in his eyes and gentle demeanour, I can see that decades of reckoning with his emotions has clearly worked.

JOURNAL PROMPTS

→ What do you do that gives your inner child freedom to express? Include activities and enabling relationships that respect your inner child and so on.

→ Do you feel guilt or shame when you let loose? If so, consider what you can say to yourself to lessen your vulnerability. For example, *I give myself permission to have fun.*

→ How can you incorporate a sense of play and fun into your daily life and work? Make a list with concrete steps on how you will achieve these things.

A playful approach to conflict is more commonly associated with parenting or infant caregiving, not adult interactions. With adulthood comes the belief that messages will be more impactful if delivered from a serious standpoint. While a humorous and playful approach isn't suited to all scenarios, it is – as supported by Morrison's practice – the perfect accompaniment for teaching and learning. The Laughter Effect can lubricate even the driest of subjects.

Both as part of my undergraduate arts degree and Master of Public Health, I had the pleasure of studying the 'sauvignon blanc' of subjects – statistics. At a US Association for Applied and Therapeutic Humor conference, jet lag got the better of me. As one presentation ended, I couldn't rouse myself from my seat and was delighted to note that the next presentation was being delivered by a professor of biostatistics.

Yawn, that would do the trick. Alas, I could not even get one of the forty winks I had planned! An emeritus professor at John Hopkins University, Ron Berk burst onto the stage timed with a blaring *Star Wars* soundtrack. His playful, witty and humorous presentation penetrated my jet-lagged mind.

That's what the Laughter Effect does. It creates a mirthful mind and primes the brain for learning. Used sensitively, humour and play improve student performance by attracting and sustaining attention, reducing anxiety, enhancing participation and increasing motivation.[12] (Especially important when statistics are involved.) Humour can initiate social interactions and conversations with challenging students, to inspire a more positive social or academic response. It may also increase interactions between students and teachers, as well as between students and peers, and draw out more introverted students.[13] Self-effacing humour illustrates to students that a teacher is comfortable making mistakes and sharing these experiences with the class. However, it should go without saying, when using humour for learning never make fun of anyone in an offensive or insensitive manner.

Sometimes a playful approach can lead to surprising and profound results. One study found playful humour enabled a fifteen-year-old to open up after three years of mutism and refusal to attend school. After some time, a mutual exchange of playful humour developed between patient and therapist.[14]

In 2021, Australian Laughter Yoga leader and educator Annie Harvey introduced the Giggle Game, comprising Laughter Yoga activities, into early learning centres. After only a couple of weeks, one girl who had not spoken during the two years she'd been there requested the 'laughter game'. The path had been paved for vocal communication in future.

In both cases, play resulting in laughter melted away the icy wall of silence. In a moment of play, transformation is possible, creating a shift in the way we experience the world. No one does this better than author and educator Dr Seuss – 'From there to here, from here to there, funny things are everywhere.' Whose counting and colour recall wasn't improved by *One Fish, Two Fish, Red Fish, Blue Fish*?

However, at times, playing with the Laughter Effect in a learning environment can quickly descend into chaos, providing the perfect scenario for a class clown to spring into action. Although humour is a near-universal trait of class clowns, many also report lower life satisfaction and less engagement with school, and with life. A clown persona can be used to mask pain and insecurity. Or as Magda Szubanski voiced in her heartfelt memoir, *Reckoning*, 'In terms of schoolyard politics, class-clown status is a form of diplomatic immunity. At last I was safe.'[15] Statistically, males more than females assume this role, with class-clown behaviour associated with having more friends but also more aggressive behaviour in the classroom.[16]

Play as therapy in challenging times

Due to the two-faced nature of a clown's personality, they don't all suit over-sized shoes and mismatched socks, like Patch Adams. Medical clowns are a special breed, playing for therapeutic gain – not just for the laugh of it – in hospital paediatric wards around the world. In Israel, a dedicated team of Dream Doctors 'operate' in every hospital. They are among first responders at the forefront of conflict, clowning from Palestinian child and their family to Jewish child and their family, from victim to perpetrator, connecting through the universal language of gibberish and nonsense. And helping to facilitate emotional release by demonstrating outward appearances are not what they seem. Behind a *kaffiyeh* (an Arab head scarf), kippah (Jewish skullcap) or painted clown face is a human being.

There are also Clowns Without Borders, whose bulbous red noses and bag of tricks spread playfulness, joy and laughter into refugee camps, conflict zones and other places where humanitarian help is needed: an increasingly vital role, with more than 1 per cent of the world's population internally displaced, refugees or asylum seekers. Of these, almost half are children.[17] Clowns Without Borders use the Laughter Effect to reduce stress and bring cheer to people of all ages in order to cope in impossibly challenging situations, when for many, all hope has been lost.

Then there is the other 'lost' world of aged care into which Elder Clowns enter residents' worlds, sharing their unique skillset of professional nonsense and enhancing positive interactions through play, song, dance, reminiscing and improvisation. I wished there'd been Elder Clowns at my dad's care facility. Alzheimer's stripped away his serious veneer. He was more in touch with his inner child in his twilight years and would have relished their playful attention. That's not the case for everyone. I recall a tight-lipped, stony-faced participant in one of the LOL sessions I facilitated, who wasted no time informing me that she would not be participating as it was all too silly (someone must have wanted her there, as permission was granted). Seated upright in a tailored suit, notebook on her lap, she exhibited an air of professionalism from a bygone life. I told her she was free to go but I sensed she was curious. Her hesitancy to connect to frivolity and play prompted my inclusion of a 'tickle monster' laugh. I encouraged everyone to wiggle their tickle monster fingers – to go through the motions of tickling – no touching. Gradually the Laughter Effect drew Madam Stern in. Surrounded by others laughing and mentally time travelling to childhood, her wrinkles softened and her face lightened up. Joy – as much as sadness – can be contagious. Fact.

My reason for choosing the tickle monster laugh was in part because tickling is an innate evolutionary behaviour. Darwin observed that it was a means of social communication in primates, and a behaviour we share not only with them but also with rats.[18] Play + tickling in rats = LOLing rats! Researchers at the University of California in San Diego constructed a 'tickle machine' and found tickling laughter stems from a different part of the brain than when evoked as an emotional response.[19] They also observed a more dramatic laughter response when tickling is directed towards bodily areas to which some animals direct their own play – under the armpits. However, whether primate, rat or human, you cannot tickle yourself. Even if you try tickling yourself in the exact same way another person tickles you, you won't laugh. Why? Because we're missing the all-important play dimension and element of *surprise*. Test it out on yourself.

Being playful need not be exclusively reserved for the fun and light-hearted moments in our lives. The challenge is playing with the Laughter Effect when it's the last thing in the world you want to do. My late father's funeral was one such occasion. Grief enveloped me. The honour of his eulogy had been bestowed on me. Because delivering a solemn remembrance would have been my undoing, the only way to curb tears was to draw on the Laughter Effect. This style was also reflective of the man my dad once was and our personal relationship, characterised by witty banter, cheeky laughter and loving reverence for one another.

I began recounting how Dad was for the large part a private man. Only a few select trusted companions would have known about his time spent in Pentridge Prison – as part of a visiting debating team. Cue the first round of laughter. Tension in the room dissipated and, more emboldened, I narrated how frustration at not becoming a surgeon was satiated later in life with a woodcarving pastime. One day he proudly showed off his latest carving – a perfect cube wrapped in a red ribbon. Customarily, we were instructed to admire from afar, but on this occasion, Dad told me to place the cube on the carpet, then walk around it. Cheekily, he congratulated me on walking around the block! More laughter. And so it went on, a waltz of tears of joy and grief.

While intoning a playful dialogue, my grief in some part was tempered, and his spirit lived on. In the following days and weeks, the approach I had taken lightened conversations with family and loved ones and helped me rise above grief's grip. My experience is supported by research about grief and humour. Mourners six months post-loss who self-reported laugh-out-loud moments were characterised by 80 per cent less anger and distress. Genuine laughers were more positive about moving forward after loss, with increased satisfaction with personal relationships.[20]

No matter your age, playing with the Laughter Effect is good for the soul, lightening the mind and reawakening your inner child. Consciously summoning play to the party releases any accumulation of laughter that's trapped internally. It builds brain capacity for creativity and learning, as well as enhancing bonding. Welcome fun back into your life. Let go of a concern for what other people think and find a way to play every day. Children do not have a Monopoly™ on this. As Irish playwright George Bernard Shaw said, 'We don't stop playing because we grow old. We grow old because we stop playing.'

7

Smile and the Whole World Smiles with You

I will never understand all the good that a simple smile
can accomplish

—Mother Teresa

Just thinking about smiling makes me smile. There is such virtue encapsulated in this simple curve. A smile is laughter's silent sister, stripping negativity in a flash while bestowing a wealth of wellbeing attributes. It's transient, yet signals social connection. Smiling is an evolutionary survival mechanism designed to increase interaction and bonding between mother and baby.

As you may recall from chapter one, Charles Darwin was so intrigued by the science of laughter, he dived headfirst into researching it. Not coincidentally, he was also the first person to examine the evolutionary nature of smiling. Through his global exploration, he noted the universal nature of smiling to be unlike verbal communication or body language, which differ between cultures. Darwin observed how muscles around the eyes are the least subject to voluntary control, explaining why faking a convincing smile can fall flat. His observations led him to conclude that human smiles paralleled the drawing back of the gums to the baring teeth in primates. He studied his own and other people's pets, and, in affirming news for dog lovers, concluded dogs do indeed smile.

The Duchenne smile

Darwin collaborated with neurologist Duchenne de Boulogne, who discovered the Duchenne smile: a smile that reaches your eyes, crumpling the corners of them into crow's feet, and is widely recognised as an expression of true happiness. Duchenne's photographic evidence led Darwin to conclude that smiling relates to happiness, whereas laughter relates to amusement. This was elucidated in Darwin's *Expression of the Emotions in Man and Animals:* 'The whole expression of a man in good spirits is exactly the opposite of that of one suffering from sorrow ... In joy the face expands, in grief it lengthens.'

Darwin's belief that these two behavioural states, smiling and laughing, which can both result in tears, stemmed from the same neurological pathways has since been discounted by modern researchers. Moreover, smiling is silent while laughter is vocalised, with different visual properties.[1]

Smiles can be broad, sincere, dramatic or spontaneous. Duchenne's name is associated with a genuine, sincere and heartfelt smile, as captured in this delightful poetic account by the man himself:

> In the newborn, the soul is bereft of all emotion and the facial expression at rest is quite neutral ... But, from the time that the infant can experience sensations and starts to register emotions, the facial muscles portray the various passions on his face. The muscles most often used by the early gymnastics of the soul became better developed and their tonic force increases proportionately.[2]

Duchenne, I romanticise, is the Father of Smiling. Without his research into smiling, who knows where we'd be? Certainly without a Duchenne smile.

Before I found out how he got his results, I was certain they stemmed from a happy and joyful activity. I pictured him sitting at a Parisian sidewalk cafe savouring a perfectly flaky croissant, conveying a warm disposition as he smiled at each and every passer-by. Alas, I was wrong.

Duchenne was a highly practical man. Initially, for his research he sourced freshly severed heads of revolutionaries, until one day he met a patient at Salpêtrière hospital in Paris, where Duchenne worked. This poor, toothless fella suffered from palsy and his face was numb to pain; he became Duchenne's muse. Over several years, he applied electrical devices to this hapless man and other subject's faces, contorting them every which way – contortions held long enough for photographs to be taken (bear in mind, this was the nineteenth century and very long exposure times were needed to counter blurry fuzz). Some sixty different facial expressions of human emotion were discovered, each depending on a dedicated group of facial muscles. Only a proportion of them translated to feel-good smiles associated with positive feelings. As for his hapless subjects – it's unlikely there were any genuine non-manipulated ones.

From Duchenne's revolutionary studies, he discovered that a smile involves the contraction of two muscles. Principally, the zygomatic major, which resides in the cheek and tugs the corners of the mouth into a smile. When combined with movement of the orbicularis oculi muscle around the eyes, the cheeks are pulled up and, in the best of ways, wrinkles form and eye brightness intensifies. (FYI, the major muscle involved in frowning, furrowing the brow, is the corrugator supercilii – another gem of a term.)

The facial feedback loop, where facial expression affects your emotional state, as observed by Darwin, explains why it's difficult to frown when looking at someone who smiles. It's those mirror neurons firing and wiring, suppressing the control we usually have on our facial muscles.

Studies on smiling

Modern researchers of positive emotion thankfully don't rely on severed heads for their work. Pre-eminent research by psychologist Paul Ekman involved compiling a taxonomy of smiles. In one project, participants across five continents were shown photographs of individuals displaying different facial expressions. They were then asked to judge what emotion they thought was being displayed in each photograph. There was majority agreement of the wide range of emotions, including pleasure, delight, cheerfulness, amusement, contentment, satisfaction, affection and flirtation. The photographs also showed embarrassment, shame, superiority and sadness.[3]

Ekman's taxonomy reflects the breadth of the human experience; a lifetime of smiling at many and varied animate or inanimate objects – a pet, a beautiful sunset, children or a partner. Ron Gutman, author of *Smile: The Astonishing Power of a Simple Act,* says more than one-third of us smile more than twenty times per day, whereas fewer than 14 per cent of us smile less than five times. Children, on the other hand, can smile as many as 400 times per day. While this statistic may not be 100 per cent accurate, there's no doubt that children smile more frequently, just as they laugh more freely.

Most smiling takes place in greetings and departures, as distinct to laughter, which is couched within conversation. Just as we have our individual laugh-print and humour-print, we also have our own smile-print. It is largely reflective of our emotional state, who we are with and what we are doing. A smile serves as a facial feedback loop and the easiest facial expression to recognise – even from a distance. Sharing a smile positively impacts both smiler and 'smile-ee', as a cocktail of happy hormones is triggered, DOSE-ing our system and instantly changing our mood.

There's more to smiling than an internal reward. In a UK study conducted by computer giant Hewlett Packard, psychologist Dr David Lewis and his team investigated a smile's bottom line. Using an electromagnetic brain scan machine and heart rate monitor, they found that, depending on whose smile you see, it can provide the same level of brain stimulation as up to 2000 chocolate bars! In this study, seeing a child's smile reaped the highest reward, equivalent to the 2000 chocolate bars. The smile of a loved one was worth about 600 chocolate treats, and the smile of a friend worth about 200.[4]

Visible changes in the brain suggest powerful emotions are triggered when we see someone important in our lives smiling at us and we smile back. Lewis interprets this as creating a 'halo' effect that helps us remember other happy events more vividly, feel more optimistic, positive and motivated. A very sweet halo. Move over retail therapy, sex therapy or sweet-tooths anonymous, a subsequent survey found that seeing a smile was more likely to create a short-term high better than sex, chocolate or shopping.

Politicians or wanna-be politicians, please take note. Many things can be faked, but *not* a smile. In this research, political smiles were voted the worst – followed by the smiles of royalty – particularly when it came to trust associated with the smile. It boils down to authenticity. A genuinely happy smile serves as a clear invitation to interact. No wonder politicians sidle up to babies in photo-ops prior to an election: if there's one thing they can usually win, it's a child's smile!

Grinning gains

Flashing your pearly whites in retail pays off – handsomely. Staff who appear to be happy and genuinely engaged in their work convey this sense of pleasure to shoppers, increasing the likelihood of a sale. I knew this to be a fact before discovering the science behind it. Personally, I'll boomerang right out of a store if I'm 'greeted' by a scowl or complete disinterest. On the other hand, when it comes to unsmiling shoppers, one particular Danish supermarket has the issue sorted. Automatic doors

CASE STUDY: Smiles per hour

Like most local government municipalities, the City of Port Phillip in
Melbourne, Australia, is heavily invested in its residents' needs, even if
that means going to somewhat unconventional means to meet them.
In 2005, Port Phillip surveyed residents on the friendliness and cohesion
of their neighbourhoods. Almost everyone expressed a desire for a more
friendly neighbourhood, noting the absence of connection with other
people in their street. Not only did people walk past each other on the
street without smiling, but they also looked down and away. Thus the
social cohesion project 'Smiles per Hour' was born.

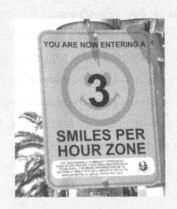

Three to four times a year, volunteers trained as neighbourhood 'Smile Spies' would walk on a defined section of a street for a fifteen-minute period with their heads held up and wearing a neutral expression. All passers-by on their side of the street were counted. People who smiled, nodded, or made any kind of positive greeting towards the volunteer when they passed them on the street were counted separately. These two numbers were converted into a percentage, amounting to the Smiles per Hour rating for that section of street. The highest rating a street could get was 100 and the lowest was zero. 'Smiles per Hour' street signs were prominently displayed, with residents encouraged to become involved as a 'Smiler', an unofficial 'Smile Trainer' or officially as a registered 'Smile Spy'. Friendly rivalry was encouraged with competitions for the informal titles of Friendliest Neighbourhood, Friendliest Street and Friendliest Shopping Centre.

Data compiled over a seven-year period showed which neighbourhoods were the 'smiliest' of them all and which could benefit from a smile infusion. It resulted in happier residents, who created a friendlier local culture, one smile at a time. Smiles per Hour was supported by the Victorian health department and Victoria Police, later crossing international borders to the Philippines, Canada and Scotland.

are programmed to only open when a smile is sensed. No smile, no shop. The net result – aisles of smiles.

Smiles are not just limited to our personal life; they also permeate our working environment and influence the nature of our interactions. When you smile, you not only appear more likeable and courteous but also more competent.[5]

In the early 2000s, a German study using MRI measured brain activity before and after injecting botox to suppress smiling muscles and found smiling stimulates our brain reward mechanism in a way not even chocolate can match. It conclusively demonstrated that irrespective of your current mood, the brain's happiness circuitry is activated when you smile.[6] And unlike calorific chocolate, frequent smiling can make you healthier, reducing stress-enhancing hormones and increasing mood-enhancing ones, which helps reduce blood pressure.

And in reverse, clinical studies in the treatment of depression found that, depending on where it's injected, botox can result in constant frowning, which may contribute to a depressed state.[7] Or, on the flip side (of a smile), the paralysis of frown muscles with botox could block this association, which may enhance positive emotions and lessen depression. However, before we further line cosmetic surgeons' pockets and book botox sessions to induce our smile, hold fire! A medicalised approach can't compete with the real deal of a natural smile.

We all make judgement calls based on first appearances. Even before we consciously choose to trust, like, avoid or dislike someone, our brain has already made an assessment. Smiling is critical to first impressions, making us look good in the eyes of others. A 2010 research project by Wayne State University in Detroit, Michigan, investigated whether smile intensity in photos impacted longevity. Using pre-1950s baseball cards of Major League players, researchers found that the span of a player's smile could predict the span of his life. Photos were divided into three categories: no smile, partial smile where only movement of muscles around the mouth engaged, or a full Duchenne smile. These were used as a measure of the intensity of a player's positivity. Players who didn't smile or smiled just with their mouth lived an average of 72.9 years, where players with beaming Duchenne smiles lived an average of almost eighty years.[8]

The last thing I want to do is tooth/smile-shame anyone. There can be reasons why people conceal their smile. Something I'm all too familiar with. Let me take you back to a younger version of myself. A Giggling Gertie if ever there was one, I had no need for an injection of anything to get a smile out of me, only for a fellow classmate to wear a grin. While I was far too shy to assume the role of class clown, I would leap at any opportunity to display my physical prowess where boys were concerned – sometimes literally. Cue the song 'Anything You Can Do (I Can Do Better)' from *Annie Get Your Gun*.

One momentous day changed the trajectory of my smile. A huge hollow cement pylon had been plonked in the school playground and naturally, come playtime, there was a race to see who could scamper to the top first. Without so much as a glimmer of doubt, I shot off, feeling ever so pleased with myself. Gleefully, I projected towards this cement giant until not only the palms of my hands and knobs of my knees made contact, but also my mouth. My first adult tooth, only recently popped to the surface, snapped off! Sent home with an airbag lip, I was swiftly escorted to the dentist, who presented Mum with two options: a white crown or a significantly cheaper (fake) silver one. Eight-year-olds didn't have an opinion in our household and Mum had an economical mindset. My tooth was swathed in silver, with promises of a white crown closer to adulthood. Any school photograph – or for that matter *any* photo – of me before that promise came to fruition is tight-lipped.

Spending many a tween year smiling expressly with my lips firmly sealed, I wonder what, if any, impact it had on my wellbeing. This is a hypothesis explored by University of California at Berkeley psychologists LeeAnne Harker and Dacher Keltner.[9] They conducted a thirty-year longitudinal study that examined photos of female students in an old yearbook to measure success and wellbeing throughout their life. They found that the women whose photos of them at age twenty-one displayed warm smiles, radiating happiness, had better health, happier marriages and expressed greater satisfaction in general with how their lives had turned out by the time they were in their fifties. They were also more likely to be more organised, content, nurturing, compassionate and sociable than females with less intense smiles. Perhaps, had I had fewer years with a silver tooth, I'd be more organised!

It also raises the question: Are the younger women happy because they're smiling, or smiling because they're happy? Or could it be as spiritual leader and poet Thich Nhat Hanh penned, 'Sometimes your joy is the source of your smile, but sometimes your smile can be the source of your joy.'

When I look at photos of myself from my childhood, there's a shyness and reservedness in the 'Silver Tooth Era'. A toothful of trauma shadowing my smile. Yet when my grin was a full complement of white, unwittingly my smile became my trademark. Decades later at a music festival, a woman I didn't recognise called out my name. It was my high school French teacher. I remarked how impressed I was that after all these years in a totally different context she remembered me. To which she replied, 'I could never have forgotten your beautiful smile.'

Not much beats a dazzling smile, which leads me to the million-dollar question: Would my husband, Danny, have fallen in love with a girl with a silver smile and would we still be married today? Is a smile a measure of the state of the union? Researchers at DePauw University in Indiana found the degree to which one smiles in photographs taken in early life predicts the likelihood that a person will divorce later in life. They first examined participants' positive expressive behaviour in college yearbook photos and then a variety of participants' photos from childhood through early adulthood. In both studies, divorce was predicted by the degree to which subjects smiled in photographs taken in childhood and early adulthood, suggesting smiling behaviour in photographs is an indication of underlying emotional dispositions, which can have direct and indirect life consequences.[10]

Stronger interpersonal bonds enhance positive emotion over the course of a lifetime, equipping people with the skills to be able to deal better with intermittent negative emotions and appraise ambiguous events more positively.[11] Smiling and laughing as a couple conveys a readiness to connect with the other – a positive emotional contagion effect playing out through one's life with a long-term partner. It's the facial equivalent of a security blanket.

What's behind a smile?

Our smile is a marker of how we feel about ourselves. A picture-perfect romantic getaway to Noosa Heads, Queensland, Danny and I went on, quickly dissolved into a nightmare over a meal. As I bit into something, my pristine white crown dislodged. All I needed was a parrot to perch on my shoulder to accessorise my new pirate look. The chip in my tooth made a dint in my confidence. Despite it being less than a quarter of my tooth, I felt ugly. I kept engagement with others to a minimum and avoided any photographs. The timid, self-conscious girl who had lay dormant for many years came to the fore. My smile had become my signature. Without it, I was anonymous. (Gratefully, my dentist restored my tooth, and my perfect smile, the day after we returned home.)

My semi-toothless adult experience (and silvery shadow of my youth) reminds me of the time when I was establishing a council-supported alternative meals program for people at risk of food insecurity. Participants needed to be vetted for eligibility. On introduction to one potential client, a man aged in his early thirties, I had to hold back my shock. Dual gums flashed back at my smile. Had we met in a dark alley, I'd have bolted in the opposite direction. But, as the saying goes, *never judge a book by its cover*. After speaking to him for a moment or two, I saw that buried under his tough demeanour lay a subdued sweetness. He hoped he'd still qualify for the program despite eating one serve of vegetables a day: potato chips! Unemployed and sleeping rough, his harsh life was worn on his face – specifically his mouth. I couldn't help but think that without the gift of teeth, his prospects were unlikely to improve as people would make assumptions about his character. I shudder to think how, in the absence of privilege, I might have stayed a pirate the rest of my life.

Exciting prospects exist for the beautiful people of the world, or so advertising companies would have us believe. We're led to believe life sucks if we don't have perfectly white, straight teeth. This helps explain cosmetic dentistry's seismic growth, including the multi-billion-dollar teeth-whitening business. After makeup, it's the largest non-surgical beauty industry. Can you name a Hollywood star with foul fangs? Over the past two decades, the number of orthodontic treatments carried out on teenagers in the United States has nearly doubled. According to a 2012 study funded by Invisalign manufacturer Align Technology, 38 per cent of Americans would rule out a second date with someone with crooked teeth, and those with straight teeth are 38 per cent more likely to be perceived as smart. Americans supposedly prefer a nice smile to clear skin and are willing to go to great lengths to get a perfect smile: 87 per cent would forego something for a year to have a nice smile for the rest of their life, even giving up dessert (39 per cent) or vacations (37 per cent).[12] While Invisalign profits from people purchasing their teeth-straightening hardware and the statistics might be mildly decayed, the story it tells is compelling.

However, not all smiles shine bright. From infancy, we're conditioned to smile to the photographic prompt, 'Cheese'. Or, as was made famous in the world's first reality TV series, *Candid Camera*: 'Smile, you're on Candid Camera.' But making a judgement call about someone's happiness from one 'happy snap' is risky business. Smiling sepia photographs of my late mother-in-law with her husband from her first marriage suggest an image of contentment – a smiling family unit. What's unseen is dysfunction, acrimony and, within months, divorce. More recently, when I 'celebrated' my second Covid-lockdown birthday in Melbourne – with Danny trapped on a film shoot interstate and my late parents absent – despite a showering of loving messages from all corners of the globe, as well as from my two beautiful boys, there was heartache behind my smile. Of course, I smiled for the camera. I smiled for the boys. I smiled for the world to see I was celebrating the blessing of life. But, as in the photos of my mother-in-law, it only depicted one frame in a much larger picture.

While smiles may not tell the whole story, they can help tell part of one. Switching on a smile was something I did during visits to my dad in aged care as language began to lose its meaning. We practised smile mirroring. Facing one another, first I'd smile, then I'd encourage him to smile, and so it would go until on occasion, like a rare diamond, his smile would sparkle into a tender laugh or chuckle. A fabulous facial work-out with the release of endorphins and the hormone of love, oxytocin. A delightful silent conversation – a 'nonversation'. A heart-to-heart soul connection, forging a bond words couldn't compete with. Naturally, I would've loved some shared conversation, even to break the monotony of the sound of my voice, but up until his dying day I felt grateful and blessed to be the beneficiary of his smile.

Even if Dad's smiles may have been devoid of situational meaning, I'm convinced they were real. Deducing true emotional state from one smile has baffled even the most esteemed scientists. Like purveyors of fine art, they've devised creative methods to sift fakes from authentic ones. In the 1980s, Fritz Strack and colleagues from the University of Würzburg in Germany asked volunteers to rate how funny cartoons were while holding a pen between their teeth (this has the effect of producing a smile without realising). Another group positioned the tip of the pen between their lips, producing a frown with no trace of a smile. Participants were told they were testing out methods to assist people with disabilities to write. Volunteers with a pen between their teeth, mimicking a smile, rated the cartoons the funniest.[13]

Please try this out for yourself.

SMILE OFF

Find a partner. Face one another. Decide who will go first at making the other person smile. The other person needs to resist smiling for as long as they can. See how long it takes to disarm them with a smile. Warning! There's a good chance it will end in laughter. Swap roles. Note how when you're smiling, you're locked into the emotional state of smiling – you won't be thinking about your stresses, you'll be too intent on sharing your smile.

Before you proclaim to each and every sour puss to simply place a pen between their teeth and they'll feel happier or even funnier, hear this – every time this experiment was replicated, it failed to match the original results. With his honour at stake, Strack repeated the experiment in 2016. To his disbelief, it flopped. The pen experiment was scribbled out until Israeli researchers modified experiment conditions – one with a video camera and one without it.[14] What transpired is that Strack, who'd received such flak, had been right after all. When participants knew they were being filmed, they didn't find the cartoons any funnier, but without the camera, Strack's original result held true, even down to the size of the effect of funniness.

Taking this idea one step further, researchers from the University of Kansas asked volunteers to bite on a pair of chopsticks: biting one end with the lips closed to produce no smile or biting along the length of the chopstick with lips apart, mimicking a standard smile. Participants were put through two stressful tasks – one a mental challenge, the other a pain induction – while chomping on said chopsticks. The researchers measured participants' heart rates and stress levels during and after the mental challenge and pain task. Those mimicking a genuine smile were less stressed and showed faster physiological recovery from the stressful tasks than those mimicking a fake smile or no smile.[15]

The pencil/chopstick trick works because it forces your face to mimic a genuine smile, engaging the muscles of the mouth, cheeks and eyes that awaken happy feelings. Contracting smile muscles changes how we perceive the world and how the world sees us, strengthening neural pathways to joy. Just don't tell your brain or it will stamp it out. Wearing a smile as opposed to a frown doesn't just make things funnier; it makes them more attractive. Participants in a Swedish study were instructed to smile or frown when exposed to positive and negative emotional pictures and then rate the pleasantness of the stimuli. Participants rated the pictures more pleasant during smiling as compared to when frowning. Although, the outcome was short-lived with no residual effects after five minutes or after one day.[16]

The endorphin effect

An important reason to work on our smile is because it enhances life satisfaction. Practising smiling for a prolonged period of time has the most impact – as demonstrated by the Swedish study – as it drugs the body with endorphins. And they're not just in our brain. Twenty types of endorphins have been discovered in the central nervous system, flowing throughout our body. They're clever little hormones, acting as neurotransmitters, transmitting electrical signals within the nervous system. Their impact on our health and immune system is substantial, modulating pain, temperature, cardiovascular regulation and respiration. Endorphins even assist gut physiology and childbirth and enhance immune system function by activating T-cells, which destroy defective or cancerous cells. They're also indirectly involved in lowering stress, improving learning, memory and motivation.

SMILING AT TRAFFIC LIGHTS

Getting hot under the collar? Traffic lights can be the best place to bring mindful awareness to your smile. The best place, because you're sitting idling with time on your hands, and that's all you need. When you're next at a traffic light, feeling agitated, connect to your breath and then welcome a smile. Smile to yourself and inhale it more deeply within, and if you're feeling bold, smile to the person in the car next to you. Having tapped into your endorphin supply, you'll be disappointed the light doesn't stay red longer.

Endorphins relax tissue so that essential antibodies can travel to affected body regions to repair and heal. When we're stressed or in shock, the endorphin flow freezes. One of my clients, 'Rachel', was diagnosed with stage four ovarian cancer. In a bid to stem her downward spiralling mood, she sought my help prior to a gruelling radiation, surgical and chemotherapy regime. It wasn't surprising that Rachel wasn't laughing or smiling much. Over the next few months, we selected practices to enhance wellness during illness, and joy amid fear and uncertainty. One such activity was an Endorphin Board – a visual representation of endorphin triggers, adapted from William Bloom's *The Endorphin Effect*. Similar to a vision board, it's a visual map of your inner smile and what makes your heart zing.

INNER SMILE ENDORPHIN BOARD

This activity is an invitation to create a visual representation of things that give you pleasure, drawing on the six major categories of endorphin triggers that make you feel good inside and out:

→ people or pets
→ places
→ activities
→ peak life experiences
→ religious or spiritual figures or symbols
→ textures, scents, sounds, tastes and colours.

Don't let this be a theoretical board. Make time to connect to these things regularly to boost mood and enhance calm and joy. Short of wall space? You can jot your triggers down on a piece of paper, fold it up and keep it in your wallet, or place highlights on sticky notes somewhere you'll see them often. Select images, such as photos or 'power' words, that you find genuinely meaningful and cause a positive response. Endorphin triggers are not static, so regularly check in and update.

The golden rule for enriching your endorphin flow:

1. Notice
2. Pause
3. Absorb

This activity can also be conducted as a mindfulness practice.

We chose an A3 cardboard sheet for her to work on. Rachel compiled images of people she loved, people who inspired her, things that made her feel good and connected her to joy: her endorphin boosters. She had samples of her hobby, ikebana – the Japanese art of flower arranging. There were inspirational quotes, too, along with swatches of her favourite colours, 'power' words and much more.

The Endorphin Board was then mounted on a wall in her bedroom. When chemo sapped her energy, Rachel had this board to gaze at and draw energy from. She could daydream into all that made her smile. On days when she felt stronger, I encouraged her to radiate this heartening sensation to loved ones who were accompanying her during this challenging time.

Initially she wasn't sure if she was doing it 'right'. I was able to reassure her that whether practising a smiling meditation or tuning into her Endorphin Board, physiological awareness grows. It might be a warm glow or fuzzy sensation, twinkle in your eye, open-heartedness or an overall softening of your body. The process of noticing, pausing and absorbing these stimuli, and switching on 'soft loving eyes', helps tap into this elixir of life. As William Bloom explains, 'The unconscious mind and the psychoneuroimmunological system cannot tell the difference between what is real and what is imagined.'[17] Happenings in the mind are real as far as the mind is concerned. Harnessing the endorphin effect changes your biochemistry.

Over the next few months, despite everything, Rachel was smiling more. Even laughter was roused, assisted by watching lighthearted movies and sitcoms. After several months, I received the best message of all. She was in remission. Neither Rachel nor I can claim the endorphin-boosting smiling practices take full credit for her recovery. However, it demonstrates how the Laughter Effect can harmoniously coexist with conventional treatments. For Rachel, integrating these techniques reawakened her inner and outer smile, optimising healing and sending this energy to her ovaries (or wherever directed) to stimulate endorphin flow. Flexing her inner smile from body to mind, and mind to body, hardwiring new neural pathways to wellbeing.

INNER SMILE MINDFULNESS PRACTICE
(FIVE TO FIFTEEN MINUTES)

1. Sitting up or lying down, close your eyes and place a smile on your face. It might help to think of a time in your life when everything was going well, or when you felt unconditionally loved.

2. Sit with this smile and note how your lips, cheeks and eyes feel as you wear this beautiful love and joy-affirming smile. Breathe the smile in and as you exhale, share it deeper into your body.

3. Now invite your smile into your heart space, filling your heart with love, a sense of ease and peace. Spend a moment or two inhaling and exhaling this smile deeper into your heart space.

4. Then direct the energy of your smile into your belly, filling it with joy, quelling any anxiety or tension. Breathing your smile in and sharing it throughout your belly and gut.

5. Now allow this smiling energy to rest wherever it's needed the most. Breathing it in and exhaling it out. Imagine the energy of your smile flowing throughout your whole body, filling every cell, tissue, fibre and muscle with this smiling energy. You're embodying a smile.

6. Know that whatever might be going on in the external world, placing a heartfelt smile on your face changes your inner world. When you're ready open your eyes and gently let go of this practice.

Superhighways of goodness are forged the more we consciously notice and appreciate the things that bring joy in our life. What *you* perceive as pleasurable and what gets your endorphins flowing is different to anyone else. If I were to ask you to bring to mind a serve of sticky date pudding, with a scoop of velvety vanilla ice cream on the side, it may result in a pleasurable response (saliva and all) or a neutral response, or – if you're gluten, dairy, date or sugar averse – a very negative response. Only *you* know what brings you pleasure and makes you smile on the inside and outside. Once you have identified your own endorphin triggers, the trick is tapping into them regularly – to stretch these pleasurable moments, allowing a deeper experience and connection. This process makes pleasurable experiences stickier, like the pudding, so our brain pays more attention to them.

At any stage of life, inner smile practices can be quite the tonic. However, you don't need to wait for a health (or other) crisis to integrate these practices into your day. It's far better to create new habits when life is smooth sailing, rather than adding another pressure when navigating choppy waters. A casualty of the Covid tsunami was our smile. Face masks impaired our connection to normalcy – our smile – particularly important if we're socially isolated, fearful or deprived of human touch. Our smiles were largely hidden. The absence of a friendly visual cue can unconsciously rewire our brains to fear and anxiety (particularly in children because of their brain's elasticity and rapid neural formation, or people prone to anxiety or depression). There was an upside, though. We were gifted an opportunity to practise smiling eyes or 'smeyes' – allowing intimacy, friendliness and sociability to rise above the cloth.

Addressing the absence of facial cues during periods of heightened stress in the pandemic prompted a mini-smile revolution in hospital staff. Kitted head-to-toe in personal protective equipment (PPE), many health workers affixed a laminated smiling portrait of themselves to their protective gear. Respiratory therapist Robertino Rodriguez, from Scripps Mercy Hospital in San Diego, described why: 'A smile goes a long way in comforting a scared patient – bringing some brightness in these dark times.' The literal act of wearing a smile lessened trauma, both in patients and staff. The brain, seeing a smile, processed it as real and cued mirror

SEROTONIN SISTER

I work from home alone. What's the best thing I can do to lift my mood?

Working from home gives you the freedom to spontaneously respond to your wellbeing needs. You could go for a walk. Tune into or add to your compilation of endorphin boosters. Take a ten-minute mindful break, adding smile breaths to your routine. Garner giggles by watching a comedy clip or listening to a funny podcast.

neuron activity, which triggered the smile's biofeedback circuit. The endorphin flow pierced PPE's facade, revealing an empathetic and caring human being.

No matter what's going on in your world – whether you're old, young, vibrant or unwell – activating your smile makes you feel better. It lightens the mind and energises the body. Cultivating an inner smile, with intention and attention, quashes an inner grudge. No matter the tone of your day, the challenges you are facing, or stage of life you're at, as clichéd as it may sound, life is better when it begins and ends with a smile. It nourishes wellbeing and strengthens connection, rippling out into the world. To quote one of my favourite philosophers, Snoopy: 'Smile and the whole world smiles at you. Slobber and they'll put you outside.'

8

Gleeful Gratitude

Be thankful for what you have, you'll end up having more.
If you concentrate on what you don't have, you will never,
ever have enough

—Oprah Winfrey

By now, you are more familiar with the multifaceted nature of the Laughter Effect. No exploration of it would be complete without adding a dimension of gratitude – one of the simplest and most potent ways to shift your life perspective and way of functioning in the world. Applying the Laughter Effect to gratitude results not only in strengthening neural pathways for all we're grateful for, but also for those associated with joy. Basking in the glow of gratitude deepens and enriches its wellbeing impact – that's the embodiment factor. It's a wonderful antidote to taking things for granted, something we've all fallen victim to at some stage in our lives. Joy-filled gratitude opens our hearts and minds to what is already there. Cicero, who was introduced in chapter one, remarked, 'A thankful heart is not only the greatest virtue, but the parent of all the other virtues.'

Gratitude and the Laughter Effect

Our days are comprised of minutes, yet how many of these can be classified as uplifting, joyous or even mildly good? Consciously layering gratitude throughout our day multiplies micro-moments of joy, so these, rather than the not-so-great moments, define its beat. This leads to greater overall happiness without needing to wait for the bigger things in life to celebrate. Otherwise, as gratitude culture expert Steven Farrugia opined, it would be like going to a footy match and holding your cheer until the final whistle. With practice, intentional gratitude, which we'll explore, becomes as unconscious as placing one foot in front of the other when we walk. It's like a torch that shines a light on the many wondrous little things in our everyday lives, no matter how seemingly small or insignificant.

When you embody gratitude, it seemingly manifests even more experiences to be grateful for. Similar to this example: Say you're in the market for a new car. You'd love a Maserati but have to settle for a red Mazda. Once you start thinking about red Mazdas, magically they appear here, they appear there, red Mazdas appear everywhere. No doubt they've been around all along, but now unconsciously you've primed your brain to pay attention. Where attention goes, energy flows. It's not so wonderful when it alerts you to the things you don't like, though. Sadly, there's a greater mental tug from an event with a negative charge than a positive one. But there's no need to get down about it – it's an evolutionary survival mechanism we owe a debt of gratitude. Otherwise, we'd risk running into the middle of a bustling highway, burning our hands on flaming hot saucepans, or binge-watching tedious programs on Netflix. The issue is when our brain constantly scours for problems to solve, even in the absence of an apparent threat. At times, we're blind to our brain's negative default, yet at other times it overpowers us and can be the source of sleepless nights. This can be explained by an in-built negativity bias playing out in our minds, or as author and neuropsychologist Rick Hanson explains, the brain is like Velcro (sticky) for the negative and Teflon (slippery) for the positive.[1]

Consider this: at the end of the day you're recounting half a dozen events or interactions. Three were positive, two were neutral and one was negative. Which one will you lie in bed thinking about? I'm guessing the negative one. Despite this interaction or event taking place in the past, your brain will continue responding in the only way it knows – sending out stress hormones mirroring the happenings in the mind's eye.

Gratitude with the Laughter Effect awakens our conscious brain to pay attention to the many habits that are so engrained we rarely notice them. Late-night gorging on chocolate, incessantly reaching for your phone, or hitting the snooze button, again and again. And again. Only when we become aware of a behaviour, habit or thought pattern can we decide to accept or change it. In doing so, we become front-seat rather than back-seat drivers in our journey.

As gratitude is not essential for survival, our brain barely pays attention. No existential threat, no flashing lights, no interest. With attention, intention and repetition (AIR), the brain begins to treat beneficial experiences with the same reverence as those linked to our survival. Otherwise, while pleasant in the moment, a beneficial thought or experience will dissipate into one of the other 6000 or so thoughts in our day. That's because these 'good' things are usually mild on the scale of intensity – a one or two out of ten – yet they are as real as negative thoughts.

Most psychological strengths, according to Hanson, are acquired from passing states or experiences of inner strength, such as gratitude, that get installed in the brain. The longer and more intense these associations, the more neurons of beneficence fire together, helping the brain journey from short-term memory into long-term storage – creating a lasting personal resource, which can be drawn on at a later date. It is a skill that can be applied to any inner strengths you'd like to develop – kindness, confidence, emotional equanimity, patience, joy, self-awareness or gratitude.

According to Hanson, spending just five or ten seconds appreciating a good experience and building associations amplifies its goodness. Adding some form of embodiment – turbocharging with a heartfelt smile or a series of smiling breaths further deepens this association. And then consciously recognising how it makes you feel and bathing body, mind and soul in its glow. That's the Laughter Effect.

Mildly beneficial experiences won't change your life but much like a cup of water is filled drop by drop, so too can your day be filled with micro-moments of joy. Reflecting on things you are thankful for helps create positive emotions, allowing you to be more content with what you already have, helping to create reserves that can be drawn on in the future to better manage threats or tension. The more focused you are on the good, the more you will smile and the more you will feel like laughing.

Regrettably, it doesn't happen overnight. Behavioural change is a process. The 'Conscious Competence' model helps us understand how the brain responds to a shift in habits. At first, we're clueless or unaware about a particular habit, giving no consideration to whether it's serving us well or otherwise – that's the beginning of the process, unconscious incompetence. Then something happens, or someone alerts us that this habit or behaviour isn't serving us well. Decision made. We will change our wily ways. Biting your fingernails is one such example. Unfortunately, you can't just click your fingers to magically inspire change; conscientious effort is required. We need to practise the new behaviour we'd like to adopt (or reject), until first we become consciously competent – still needing to think about what we're doing and then, with repetition, becoming unconsciously competent, where we don't think about this habit or behaviour, we just do it.

This same theory can be applied to habitual thoughts or passing emotional states, like gratitude. Without having an MRI, we can monitor changes in our brain, in the comfort of our own home.

TEN FINGER MINDFUL APPRECIATION PRACTICE

This is a fun activity to introduce to children. Each day, counting
with each finger on your hands, call to mind ten things you're
grateful for. If you do this practice every day there may be repetition
but that's okay. They really add up! Ten things a day, seventy things
a week, 280 things a month, etc. This is a great way to hardwire
neural pathways to goodness.

Grow gratitude

Here's a technique to grow gratitude. If you're a watch wearer, for the
next week or so, each day place it on your other wrist. If you don't wear
a watch, place any item of jewellery on your other wrist or hand, or
brush your hair or teeth with your non-dominant hand. Choose any
habit you do one way and try doing it another. Initially your brain will
have a mild hissy fit and throw lots of resistance your way. *This takes too
long. Why would she make me do this? This is so frustrating. Nup, I don't
want to do this.* After a few days, resistance will soften, and within a week
or so, most likely you'll place your watch on the other hand or reach
for your toothbrush with your non-dominant hand without so much
as a thought.

With practise, activities can become second nature – dirty clothes
usually tossed on the floor can make the huge leap into the washing
basket; swallowing your food before you talk as opposed to spraying it
out of your mouth; appreciating what your partner does for you rather
than criticising their every flaw. That's where the rewiring comes in. It's
the equivalent of taking your brain to the gym – bicep curls for positive
neuroplasticity.

An attitude of gratitude feeds an upward cycle of positive emotion. Honing our internal radar to grasp opportunities that may present

to us. Leaning into the good, which means leaning away from the not so good. Not even the most talented dancer can simultaneously lean in two directions!

. . . .

Practising gratitude is far easier when life is cruisy, but when things are not going so well – during grief or loss, financial stress, relationship tension or illness – it can seem about as removed as a hot summer's day in mid-winter. I realised this three days after my bowel resection, when I received the wonderful news that the cancer had not spread. To say I was relieved would be an understatement; I was overwhelmed with gratitude. However, it was as if my body didn't know what to do with it. That only came with the outpouring in black pencil on the white hospital placemat as I focused my attention on the many things and people I was grateful for: my body for graciously supporting me during the five-hour surgical onslaught; having the operation in a world-class hospital; my loving family and friends. I distilled moments of gratitude until I was embodying it at both a neural and cellular level. The Laughter Effect's uplifting energy flooding every cell, tissue and muscle. The more I was thankful for, the more expansive the feeling. A high without the need for a morphine top-up.

From that moment, I made a commitment to cultivate a thankful heart. First, dipping my toe in the gratitude well, and then fully immersing. I was inspired by the founder of Positive Psychology, Professor Martin Seligman, whose research into daily recounting of Three Good Things 'demonstrated long-lasting effects on depression and happiness'.[2] Three Good Things involves making a mental or written stocktake of back-to-basics 'good things' often taken for granted. On the cusp of sleep, rather than counting sheep, I'd recount three things that went well in my day: blessings or gestures of kindness I observed or received. Lost in these moments, leaning into the good, I received a mini respite from past concerns or future worries.

SEROTONIN SISTER

I've recently lost my partner of forty years and there are some days I can't even find one thing I'm grateful for. Feeling grateful feels inauthentic. What can I do?

Once we allow our mind to journey from the gaping hole that grief leaves behind, we can begin to lean into the many good things in our day. Downsize what you're grateful for into little bites – your comfortable bed, a soothing hot shower, or beautiful memories you shared with your loved one – rather than trying to identify huge chunks. Otherwise, turn inwards, to qualities you appreciate about yourself that are helping you through this challenging time.

On days when my mood was low and anxiety high my resistance would peak and I'd wonder how I'd come up with three *whole* things. Yet once the gratitude juices began flowing, they were hard to stop. Leaning into the good feels good. Even a little addictive, explained in part by the release of dopamine, as a connection is made between the behaviour and feeling fab. The more expansive the gratitude practice, the more hits of dopamine. Until we become drunk on gratitude.

A GRATITUDE SMILING BODY SCAN

1. Make yourself comfortable. Take a deep breath in and out, repeat. With each breath, surrender a little more. Every day your breath is there for you and has been for every moment in your life. Without telling it to do so, it just breathes. Offer gratitude for your breath. Smile into your breath and exhale deeply.

2. Now bring your attention to your face. We can be very judgemental about our faces. Bring awareness to your cheeks, to your lips, your nose. Become aware of your eyes and eyebrows. Try not to get lost in any judgements – just notice. Bring awareness to your neck and the back of your head. Now to your whole head. Feel a sense of gratitude for your whole face and head with a heartfelt smile. Breathe this sense of gratitude in, and as you exhale, share this gratitude from your face deeper into the body.

3. Now bring your awareness to your shoulders, your upper arms, elbows, lower arms, wrists, the palms of your hands, the back of your hands and your fingers. Invite a sense of gratitude. Inhale this feeling of gratitude, and as you exhale, share gratitude with a heartfelt smile for your arms for all they do – from your shoulders to your fingertips. Express gratitude with a smile, and as you exhale, share this smile with your shoulders, arms and hands.

4.   Shift your awareness to your chest, your solar plexus, belly, hips and pelvic area. Now your torso and lower back, your middle back, your upper back. Inhale a feeling of gratitude for this whole area, and as you exhale, share this feeling deeper within. Bring a smile to your face, and as you exhale, share this smile with the front and back of your chest, solar plexus, belly, hips and torso.

5.   Repeat this exercise and bring awareness to your thighs, fronts and back of your knees, your lower legs, ankles, heels, soles of your feet and toes.

6.   Now bring awareness to your whole body, from the top of your head to the tips of your toes. Feel your breath moving in and out of your body. Thank it for all it does. How it supports and carries you through life. How it enables you to touch and feel, to see and smell, to hear and taste, to live and love. With each inhalation the feeling of gratitude grows, and each exhalation allows it to reset each cell of your body.

7.   Your body is always with you, as is the feeling of gratitude. You don't need a special invitation to feel gratitude towards any of your body parts. Practise thanking them. The parts you love, the parts you don't especially like, those that work hard for you, and even the ones that seemingly serve no purpose whatsoever. Your body always tries to do its best.

8.   Gently let go of this practice and allow your eyes to float open.

How gratitude benefits the body

Gratitude fuels our body's in-built antidepressant, serotonin, which kicks in when we reflect on past significant achievements or things that have gone well in our life. Or so we thought. New research by Dr Joe

Dispenza – teacher, chiropractor, researcher and author – has revealed we can also be future grateful. We can connect to the emotion of gratitude even before an actual event has happened. Doing so tricks our body into believing this future event is happening in the present moment or has already happened. This provides an opportunity for both mind and body to mentally experience this grateful state before physically tasting its fruits. The choice is ours – to daydream or nightmare. Either way, the body responds in kind.

Using heart rate variability and brain scans, Dispenza's research revealed trading emotions like anger and fear, frustration or impatience, two or three times a day for fifteen minutes to feel gratitude results in 50 per cent more chemical immunoglobulin A (IgA) being produced – the body's natural 'flu shot'. Embodying elevated heart-centred emotions like love, joy or gratitude in your inner environment signals the switch from the sympathetic to the parasympathetic nervous system. With fewer stress hormones circling like sharks and more hormones associated with wellbeing, the level of threat in the external environment is downgraded from hazardous to harmless, enhancing the capacity for healing and strengthening our immune system.

Practising gratitude changes the heart's rhythm and the messages it sends to the brain, enacting uplifting emotion and signalling the autonomic nervous system to take a break from fear. Activating the energy of the Laughter Effect and sinking into a grateful smile lets our body know it's receiving emotions. This results in heartbeat coherence, or when shared, swelling gratitude in another's heart. And from there, it extends out into the broader energy sphere.

Fifteen minutes might sound onerous, yet you can embrace gratitude when you've just woken up, to set the emotional tone of your day and anchor the energy of gratitude into your being. With a gentle smile in tow, bring to mind three or more things you appreciate about yourself or others. Then throughout your day, graze on gratitude. Intentionally seek and lean into moments of goodness – at meals, during meditation, when you're out walking, or journaling. Grow the goodness that's already there. Consequently, you'll propel a move towards living gratefully, as opposed to merely having grateful experiences.

GRATITUDE LETTER TO YOURSELF

Write yourself a letter of gratitude, thanking you for all you do. Allow a sensation of heartfelt gratitude to bathe your body as you're writing. Use this as an opportunity to embrace any self-perceived imperfections, perhaps the shape of your nose or scars (emotional or physical) you bear. Here is an example for you to expand upon and direct your gratitude, genuinely and abundantly.

To my dear self,

Thanks for not giving up on me, even when I gave up on you.
Thanks for a lifetime of seeing, hearing, feeling, for my heartbeat.
Thanks for all the experiences you've showered me with, even if at the time I found them difficult to accept.
Thanks for my friendships, family and acquaintances, for all the support in my life.
Thank you for accepting the whole of me and refraining from judgement.
Thank you for accompanying me through life imparting your infinite wisdom even when I did not want to hear it.

In loving appreciation and gratitude,
Me xox

Being grateful pays off in weird and wonderful ways. Research conducted at Northeastern University, Massachusetts, asked 105 undergraduate students to complete a specific task on a computer. The computer was rigged to break down when they were close to completion. When the glitch was fixed, participants were told they'd need to start over. Actors engaged as IT 'geeks' were called in to solve the problem. One can only imagine the first question they asked participants was, 'Have you tried turning it off and on again?' Then, at the press of one button, the computer was revived and the task they'd been working on was saved. Most study participants reported feeling gratitude towards the actor. Over the next three weeks, their gratitude levels were measured. Students who felt more gratitude during the computer meltdown exercise also felt more grateful throughout their week. When it came to being remunerated for their time in the study, students who demonstrated more gratitude were happy to hold out for a higher amount of cash at a later date, as opposed to the less grateful participants who favoured a smaller amount of cash on the spot.[3]

Gratitude practices for individuals

Practising gratitude promotes resilience and helps to guard against the negative impact of burnout, which is why it's consistently on my go-to list as a way to enrich clients' lives. One of my clients, 'Steve', was a burnt-out middle manager on extended leave from a large IT firm. He was curious to give positivity resilience coaching a go, to lift him out of his funk. I wasn't sure how he'd respond to my recommendation of a daily gratitude practice. Perhaps it lacked the gravitas he'd anticipated. However, intuitively I believed it would be fundamental in reviving his depleted spirit.

The first step was to expand his understanding of gratitude, from the simplistic notion of thanks to an expanded notion of appreciation for what gives life meaning and value. I highlighted one of the most tested and effective gratitude-boosting techniques – a gratitude journal. (We'll discuss more about journaling in chapter ten). Mindful of his stress levels, I relayed a study where one group of cardio patients was instructed to keep a gratitude journal for eight weeks, and to write about two or three things they were grateful for – their partners or children, pets, friends, jobs – most days of the week. The other group followed clinical recommendations alone. At the end of the study, patients who kept gratitude journals exhibited a better mood, better sleep, less fatigue and other factors pertaining to cardiac health.[4] Two months later they were retested. Those who had continued writing in their journals displayed lower levels of inflammation and improved heart rhythm with a decrease in heart disease risk.

Another casualty of Steve's burnout was his relationships with his nearest and dearest. It's hard giving emotionally to others when you're in the red. According to Robert Emmons, psychology professor and gratitude researcher at the University of California, gratitude strengthens relationships because it requires us to see how we've been supported and affirmed by other people. And demonstrating our gratitude to loved ones makes them feel good, which in turn make us feel good. It was time for Steve to let his loved ones know how much he valued them, to convey he was not taking their love or support for granted. He needed to activate the Laughter Effect, fuelling a reciprocal upward spiral of positive behaviour.

My sessions with Steve were informed by an understanding that grateful people are also more likely to feel optimistic, both about their own lives and the world around them. They're also more inclined towards flexible thinking than naysayers. One study revealed a 5 to 15 per cent increase in optimism following a gratitude journaling practice.[5] The more helpless Steve had become, the more his optimism had whittled away. Developing a positive outlook for the future was key to dredging him out of his burnt-out state. By the end of our initial session, he told me he was up for the gratitude challenge. It was the perfect time to present him with homework tasks for the week ahead – to begin wearing his wristwatch on the other hand and compile a gratitude journal, expanding on the Three Good Things exercise.

Over a couple of months, Steve's transformation was remarkable and clearly linked to his dedicated gratitude practice. He'd successfully reprogrammed his brain to tone down negativity by regularly and deeply homing into goodness in his day. His neural pathways towards positivity were emboldened and he was feeling considerably more optimistic about his relationships, prospects for returning to work, and life in general. He reported smiling more both inwardly and outwardly. Years later I bumped into him on the street. Excitedly he pointed to his watch. He was still wearing it on his other wrist. I explained I hadn't expected him to continue this practice, but he said he liked a visible reminder to begin every day with a grateful mind. Now back in the workforce, Steve told me how he eagerly sought opportunities to share gratitude with his co-workers, celebrating and appreciating the many small wins, achievements and progress within his team.

WRITE A GRATITUDE JOURNAL

Why don't you give gratitude journaling a go? Capture the day's goodness by writing down three things that went well in your day and provide an explanation for why they went well. The items you recall can be relatively small in importance (I had a lovely catch-up with . . .) or relatively large (I landed my dream job). Write down what happened in as much detail as possible, including what you did or said and, if others were involved, what they did or said. Note how this event made you feel at the time and how it made you feel later. Did you smile on the inside and/or outside? If you navigate towards negative feelings, refocus your mind on the good event and allow the positive feelings to flow. Note where in your body you feel the sensation of gratitude, smile into it, and allow the energy of the Laughter Effect to soak more deeply within. This practice is a great way to train your brain to notice and absorb the good in your day. In time you won't need to go into as much detail to connect to your gratitude.

Grateful workplaces

Workplaces can be a major contributor to personal stress. We've seen how the Laughter Effect can enhance social, emotional and psychological wellbeing by drawing on humour, laughter and play – so too can an institutional culture of gratitude. However, research suggests people are less likely to feel or express gratitude at work than any other place, with some employees hesitant to express thanks fearing it could be seen as a sign of weakness, or that it might inadvertently embarrass their colleagues.[6] Factoring in the hours spent at work over a lifetime, this is a setting crying out for gratitude's gracious and nurturing touch.

Employing gratitude at work can have a significant positive impact on staff's mental health, stress and the rate of turnover. It helps inspire a relational as opposed to purely transactional work environment and is a potent way of conveying to employees and colleagues that they're valued. Finding things to be grateful for at work, even in stressful jobs, can help protect staff from the negative side effects of their job.[7] It works best when leadership and management styles build a persistent gratitude habit and don't leave it to chance, with regular gratitude helping to lessen burnout. It then filters top down to all levels of an organisation, no matter the size or setting – a school, local government, corporate workplace or community organisation. Demonstrating appreciation serves to unite and motivate in ways money cannot compete, resulting in a collective mindset of thankfulness.

Gratitude in the workplace is also contagious – the more it's expressed and amplified throughout an organisation, the more it's reciprocated among employees. It's a means of authentically creating ripples of goodness, lauding pro-social, we-centric behaviour, producing results that CEOs and managers are after – enhanced performance, productivity and staff retention. The ripple effect of gratitude is far superior if it's embedded into the core values of an organisation, rather than only expressing it on World Gratitude Day.

As an extension of the Laughter Yoga (LOL) pilot I ran in the aged care facilities, I organised a training program for staff, to equip them with the skills they'd need to introduce laughter activities into their workplace. An aged care facility I'd yet to visit offered to host one of the training sessions. A charming staff member showed me around before I began formal training. The lightness and joviality in the corridors immediately struck me. Smiles and chatter echoed between staff and residents. Far more so than other facilities I'd visited. My tour culminated with a quick cuppa in the staff kitchen and dining room before the formal training began. Staring me in the face, almost one entire wall was dotted with colourful sticky notes – a 'Wall of Appreciation', bearing messages of appreciation for their colleagues. Now the atmosphere made sense. This wall served as a visual prompt, motivating staff to perform better at work, and at a deeper level, to become enriched human beings.

Positive qualities were celebrated, as opposed to so many other workplaces where there's a tendency for negative ones to be magnified. At this facility, compliments and other gestures of appreciation were encouraged, resulting in seemingly happier, more satisfied employees. However, you don't have to build a wall. There are many ways individuals and teams can embed a culture of gratitude.

. . . .

Seek opportunities to satisfy your altruistic side by volunteering. Tap into the helper's high, sparking a host of wellbeing benefits. Generate a *double good* – creating a biofeedback cycle of gratitude between giver and recipient. As Scottish novelist and playwright Sir James Matthew Barrie, creator of *Peter Pan*, articulated in the early nineteenth century, 'Those who bring sunshine to the lives of others cannot keep it from themselves.'

Become fluent in the language of gratitude

It also pays to speak the language of gratitude – to become fluent in abundance, blessings and gifts lingo. The Laughter Effect develops fluency in gratitude by not solely going through the *motion* of it, but also going through the *emotion* of it. It helps us fall in love with the life we already have. To recognise the qualities that enrich our existence and the even larger miracle of being alive.

AFFIRM YOUR GRATITUDE

This is one of my favourites.

> *I am grateful for this moment*
> *I am grateful for every breath*
> *I am grateful for all my blessings*
> *I am grateful for my life.*

Once you've composed your affirmation, turbocharge these words with a whole body smile and repeat regularly.

When you take time to bathe in the energy of gratitude, you'll feel more optimistic and joyful. Gravitating towards gratitude makes life more rewarding. The more you anchor yourself to a present moment of goodness and allow its potency to soak in, the more you'll begin smiling on the inside. That's the Laughter Effect. With a heart and mind full of gratefulness, you'll feel better within yourself and have more to offer others. It will grow the good in them, too, widening ripples seen and unseen. If ever you harbour an ounce of doubt, pause and ask yourself, *In this moment, what can I be grateful for?* Because there is always something to be grateful for. As Eckhart Tolle affirmed, 'Acknowledging the good that you already have in your life is the foundation for all abundance.'

CASE STUDY: A recipe for gratitude soup

In the 1960s, Andy Warhol's artistic works of cans made Campbell's Soup a household name. And in 2001, when Douglas Conant took over as president and CEO of Campbell's Soup, he added another masterful stroke. At the time, finances were dire. Employees were disheartened, trust was low and layoffs were commonplace. Of all the major food companies in the world, it earnt the label of the lowest-performing – one it was desperate to shed. The environment was so toxic that a Gallup manager described employee engagement as 'among the worst [he had] ever seen among the Fortune 500'.[8]

Conant is a people's person, so one of his priorities was to enhance employee engagement. Literally walking the talk, he wore a pedometer on his belt, aiming for 10,000 steps a day to meaningfully interact with as many employees as possible. It didn't matter whether he was at the New Jersey headquarters or another production plant in the world, he'd meet and greet employees from maintenance staff to executives. Additionally, each day he handwrote up to twenty notes a day to employees, celebrating their successes and specific contributions. This amounted to more than 30,000 notes in the ten years of his leadership, and there were only 20,000 employees. One can only imagine the sea of smiles generated from these handwritten encapsulations of 'I see you', 'I celebrate you', 'I value you'.

Conant and his team achieved extraordinary results. Sales and earnings were on the upswing. Business was flourishing and employee engagement was at world-class level. His letters of appreciation paid off in ways he never anticipated when, in 2009, he was in a serious car accident. He was inundated with get-well notes from all reaches of the Campbell's Soup world.

'As my wife and I sat and read them in the hospital room, I could feel them helping to speed my recovery. The blessings of their notes reminded me that the more supportive feedback you give to others, the more you may very well receive in return.'[9]

Drawing on over thirty years in his career, Conant has divulged his secret recipe for gratitude based on these three rules:

1. Make a personal connection early on. Your associates can tell when you are being direct, sincere and authentic. When you are, you establish trust. When you aren't, you don't. A powerful tool for relationship-building is sharing your background, values, leadership philosophy, expectations and even favourite quotes with the people you meet with. Then ask them to share something with you.

2. Look for opportunities to celebrate. Conant and his executive assistants spent thirty to sixty minutes a day scanning mail and their internal website looking for news of people who'd made a difference at Campbell's.

3. Get out your pen. Let people know you're paying attention and celebrating their accomplishments. Seek out opportunities to write to people who partner and collaborate with your company and help bring you success. Writing handwritten notes may seem like a waste of time, but in Conant's experience they build goodwill and lead to higher productivity.[10]

9

Self-Compassion with
a Smile

*If I am not for myself, who will be for me? If I am not for others,
what am I? And if not now, when?*

—Rabbi Hillel

The Laughter Effect provides a shield to some of the mental health challenges posed by a world obsessed with perfection. Self-compassion with
a smile is associated with numerous wellbeing benefits, including higher
levels of positivity, optimism, happiness and lower levels of anxiety and
depression. These are skills I wish I'd grown up with. To be able to lovingly smile at and embrace the whole of me. However, I have a hereditary
condition. It's called 'giving-itis'. You may have heard of it before. Perhaps you have a form of it yourself. This syndrome ranges from a chronic
need to do good, to a milder condition where you passively, rather than
actively, seek to do good. Giving to others at the expense of yourself is
a fundamental component. It is underpinned by a sound moral value:
treating others as you would like to be treated. Sage advice on the face of
it, yet too often one-sided. If only we treated *ourselves* as we did others.

I'm certain giving-itis is a genetic condition that can be traced back
multiple generations in my family tree. I inherited it from both my
maternal and paternal genes, particularly from the female lineage. It was

reinforced every evening at dinner when I was growing up. My mum would serve everyone else first and be seemingly content with whatever remained, even if that was the chicken's carcass. She was a chronic 'do-gooder' and we literally digested the fruits of her selflessness for years as she trialled all the recipes in the fundraising cookbook she coordinated for our local synagogue. Mum's goodness overflowed into many roles, including decades as an active member of B'nai B'rith (the Jewish equivalent to Rotary). Life was about serving and enriching the lives of others, and the thought of applying that same degree of reverence to oneself was unheard of.

Without a role model, it's no surprise that becoming more self-compassionate has been one of my greatest hurdles. Please note, I wrote *becoming* as opposed to *being*. Becoming more self-compassionate is an ongoing process. As I entered adulthood, inner or self-compassion didn't come close to rivalling other self-care practices, such as healthy eating and exercise. I was 'smart' enough to know there were far more significant influences on my wellbeing than being 'lovey-dovey' to myself. But I would have been spared a lot of pain had I realised the importance of self-compassion. When our inner sense of love or self-worth falters, we fly into other people's storms, take everything personally and become a victim of their bad weather. A self-compassionate heart-set not only protects us from this, but it also guards us from our own turbulence.

Something I've fallen foul to many a time is sinking while convincing myself I was swimming. All those years ago after my bowel cancer operations when meals lovingly prepared by friends ran out, I'd hobble to the stove to prepare a home-cooked meal for the family. I know what you're thinking. Why didn't I just ask for more help? Or order takeaway? Because that would have taken a degree of self-compassion I did not possess. Far better to suffer within than run the risk of inconveniencing someone else, or cough up funds for something I could prepare more cheaply. How could I become more self-compassionate when I didn't even know it was a thing?

HOW COMPASSIONATE ARE YOU?

Take a moment to rate yourself on a scale between one and ten on how compassionate you are to others: one is not compassionate at all and ten is super-compassionate. Now rate your level of self-compassion, using the same scale, one to ten. How similar or different is each rating to the other?

Here's a personal fact about me. I have highly attuned psychic abilities ... and I am sensing that if you are a woman reading this, you're more compassionate to others than to yourself. Am I right? If so, you're in good company. Research shows, on average, women have significantly more compassion for others than men, but less compassion for themselves. Statistically, women feel less entitled to meet their own needs and are instead valued for self-sacrifice and meeting the needs of others.[1] Clearly a result of societal structures and the maternal role women have played for thousands of years, and today we still live with the consequences. However, it does not suggest this is true of all women or men.

If self-compassion isn't learnt from family or friendship circles, where does it come from? It's not as if we need to pass a self-compassion exam to graduate from high school. While self-compassion has yet to be branded a critical life skill, it most certainly deserves to be. In my case, professional curiosity rather than a personal quest enabled me to stumble upon self-compassion as a concept and technique to enhance wellbeing.

Self-esteem versus self-compassion

At the annual Happiness and Its Causes conference, educational psychology associate professor Kristin Neff, from the University of Texas in Austin, spelt out the three core components of self-compassion – kindness, common humanity and holding painful feelings in mindful awareness. Up until that conference, my understanding of self-compassion had been rudimentary, at best. Neff demystified some of the more common misperceptions of self-compassion, such as it in no way relates to self-indulgence or self-esteem. Unlike self-esteem, which tends to involve evaluating oneself in comparison with others, self-compassion is non-evaluative. It's an internal resilience enabling you to bounce forward from hardship and suffering without falling too far. It's a starting point when things are tough – not where you stop. It's when a sense of care is lovingly nurtured after a setback. An empowering thought. Even if you don't feel particularly good about yourself, are experiencing pain or going through a challenging time, you can still be compassionate towards yourself, just as you would demonstrate compassion towards someone else going through something similar, regardless of whether you fully approve of their actions or words or appreciate their situation.

Neff spoke of self-compassion being a way of positively relating to oneself. Mitigating inner turmoil arising from inner self-judgement and self-criticism. I found myself nodding at her explanation of how it can be easier to be the self-critic rather than the vulnerable voice who knows they've messed up. That self-compassion is an attitude involving treating oneself with warmth and understanding in difficult times and recognising that making mistakes is part of being human.

I was comfortably sat back in my seat, furiously taking notes, when it came time to put theory into practice. A short three-part self-compassion break. Five minutes of inner 'squeam'. (I'm aware the full word is squeamish, but I was 'squeaming' – inwardly screaming squeamishness.) First, Neff invited us to bring to mind a little suffering. Nothing huge. On mentioning 'suffering', like a dog's hackles, my resistance pricked, made all the worse by my inner voice chiding me for being so resistant. 'Suffering' seemed a little extreme. I wasn't *suffering*. I felt that term should be reserved for impoverished people, domestic violence victim-survivors or homeless people. Not a middle-aged privileged white female.

Neff invited us to bring a quality of mindfulness to witness our pain or suffering from a more detached perspective. Bringing to mind this 'suffering', name it and let go of judgement. Hold on a second, *judgement* was a standard I held dear. That's how I remained accountable to myself. I feared if I released judgement, I would be hollow on the inside. Yet here I was being asked to take a step back and mindfully notice, without judgement; to turn, with loving awareness, towards my suffering or pain.

Her words pierced my protective shield, bypassing my mind and shooting directly to my heart. My inner demons panicked. They were exposed. Naked. I was fearful they could be seen by the thousand or so other people in the auditorium. Gulp. It dawned on me then and there: I excelled in compassion for others, but self-compassion – not so much.

With the second step, inviting a sense of common humanity to my situation, I began decompressing. We all fail, make mistakes and face serious life challenges. No one is perfect or leads perfect lives. We all suffer, face illness, lose people we love ... Phew, perhaps I wasn't such a failure. We're all *perfectly imperfect*.

To the third step – inviting self-kindness. This is about being caring and understanding to oneself rather than being harshly critical for any perceived personal shortcomings. To offer ourselves warmth and unconditional acceptance with a gentle embrace or soothing words. All this felt a little uncomfortable until – and I am sure Neff was reading my mind – she suggested we might like to call to mind words of comfort or soothing we'd offer a loved one in a similar circumstance. Once we found the right words, we could draw on this language for ourselves.

Self-compassion versus self-pity

After Dr Neff's presentation, I was left considering that if suffering comes from inner self-judgement and self-criticism, then without a doubt I had experienced *multiple* moments of suffering; I'd just never acknowledged them as such, gritting my teeth and continuing blindly on. One example is painfully breastfeeding my first-born when a matronly nurse advised that 'whether through cracked nipples or engorged breasts, you continue to breastfeed'. I lapped up her advice. Welcome to motherhood. Chin up. Milk away! Only after a couple of agonising weeks, when inflammatory thrush got the better of me, did I begin treatment to quell symptoms and pain. I never thought there was a way to express how dismal I was feeling without sounding like a *woe is me* victim. Motherhood was a gift and blessing; how could I complain when I'd chosen to become a mum, given birth in a world-class hospital and had a supportive and loving family? I had confused self-compassion with self-pity. Offering compassion to myself in my role as a new mum was as foreign to me as my newborn son's understanding he was a birthed human being. Unconditional love was something I'd indubitably bathe him in, but not myself.

Humans are hardwired to survive. When circumstances become stressful, we go into fix-it mode, managing the best way we can. We rarely take the time to pause and validate how difficult a situation might be or encourage or motivate ourselves in a self-soothing fashion. Receiving care or support from an external source can feel more natural than when it's self-directed as it's more consistent with the care model we're accustomed to. We'll go to great lengths to avoid feeling awkward or uncomfortable, even if ironically it's 'only' to ourselves. However, outsourcing care is not always the solution. Besides, why wait for what we can provide ourselves 24/7 if we so choose.

Practise what you preach

After my impactful introduction to self-compassion with Kristen Neff, I began putting it into practice. I took baby steps, smiling lovingly and without judgement at myself in the mirror. Endeavouring to avoid the cringe. Greeting myself, eye to eye with acceptance as I would a loved one.

One pimple does not destroy a beautiful face! I placed Post-it notes decorated with love hearts at my bedside, desk or sneakily positioned in a place only I would see, to avoid 'why are those notes everywhere, Mum?' I'd end the day with a positive affirmation: *I am beautiful, I am doing a great job, I love myself.* I wish I could say it was easy, that it didn't feel forced and that these words effortlessly flowed from within, without silently gagging. I'd remind myself I was becoming more compassionate, that it was a process. Just like everyone else, I was a work in progress. Some avenues to inner compassion came easier. Smiling or lovingly laughing at myself about encounters that hadn't gone as smoothly as I'd wished were a cinch. I tried to catch myself in a nurturing mood before lurching into self-critical or blaming mode. Comforting myself, saying it was okay, I was okay, I was more than okay, most definitely took a little getting used to.

In my daily meditations, I would embrace my emotional needs through words, feelings, touch or mantra. Guided by my heart, I began feeling more joy, contentment and overall positivity – about myself and life in general. It was a milestone in being able to see and feel the positive, no matter what kind of day I'd had.

As my confidence grew, self-compassion breaks became a regular fixture for my individual and corporate clients. No matter the audience, I'd pose the question about how compassionate they were versus how self-compassionate. Time and again, people would rate admirably high in compassion but dismally in self-compassion. I'd iterate how it wasn't about robbing from one pot to give to another. That being kind and non-judgemental towards the self was good practice for treating others compassionately. No matter how educated the crowd, not only were peoples' inner dialogues unsupportive, in many instances they were outright bullies. A pattern was also seemingly emerging: the more caring, personally and/or professionally, the lower the self-compassion.

Similar to my first experience with Kristen Neff, after self-compassion breaks there was often awkward silence, gently requiring me to coax people back from their internal brink. A critical care worker at a major hospital in Melbourne was startled that his inner voice had been drowned out by his reproving father's. Others in the nursing profession berated themselves for perceived failures, and teachers were quick to brand themselves as silly or stupid. Like me, they were either victims of being parented in a certain way or received modelling from a school of thought that lauded being tough and harsh as a motivator for learning, erroneously believing it would make them more resilient. Rather than being lovingly accepted and embraced for weaknesses as well as strengths, messages of not being good enough and a sense of failure permeated their core.

The way we learn as children sets the scene for learning as adults. If you were used to a firm hand and callous voice motivating you as a child, there's a good chance you'll mirror this behaviour later in life. If not to your own children, then to yourself. Kindness may appear weak; however, it's amazing how far people can soar on its wings.

One program I facilitate lays bare our learnt 'defective' messaging system. An exercise where participants compile a list: ten things I don't like about myself. Easy, you think. But here's the twist. That list is swapped with the person sitting opposite who reads, out loud, the list of imperfection or failures. Ouch!

- 'I hate the way I look'

- 'I feel like a fake'

- 'I always mess up'

- 'I'm a crappy mother'

- 'I'm a bad son'

- 'I'm stupid'

- 'I'm not especially loveable'

Who needs enemies when we have ourselves? I don't leave the exercise here, with participants sucked into a gaping hole of self-loathing. The next task is about listing ten complimentary traits. There's no need to swap these. In some regards, it's a more challenging exercise but with considerably less chance of squirming.

Self-compassion or self-comparison?

I have wondered how much of the inequity between inner and outer compassion can be blamed on society's lack of respect for self-compassion. Social media is awash with hashtags such as #Fail! #Loser #Instaloser, and dominated by visions of perfection. Perfect teeth, perfect partner, perfect house, perfect car, perfect job, perfect breasts. It makes for a perfect noose! With a perfectionist mindset, we can never be enough. To avoid putting yourself in a situation where you might fail – for example, not receiving the desired number of likes – you don't take the risk. You can't fail if you don't try, and if you don't try, your inner demons are safe and sound.

Perfectionism can be viewed as self-oriented perfectionism (excessively high personal expectations), socially prescribed perfectionism (excessively high social expectations) and other-oriented perfectionism (excessively high expectations of others).[2] Socially prescribed perfectionism has been found the most destructive on mental health. If only we could embrace the ancient Japanese art principle of *kintsugi* in our lives – a beautiful tradition where broken pottery is pieced together with gold, creating a stronger and even more beautiful art piece, despite its 'flaws'.

A more self-compassionate approach is also a potent antidote for our predilection for 'comparisonitis' – a quasi-subset of perfectionism. We can never truly shine as long as we are measuring against someone's shadow. Compared to higher self-esteem, greater inner compassion results in a stronger negative association with social comparison, public self-consciousness, self-rumination, anger and a fixation on a definite conclusion.[3] Where failures can be viewed as a part of life and an opportunity for learning. Self-compassion loosens the grip on negativity by generating positive emotion towards the self and distancing labels of 'good' or 'bad'.

Social psychologists at the University of California, Berkeley, conducted a series of experiments that proved the theory that self-compassion motivates people to improve personal weaknesses, moral transgressions and test performance. Far from making you lazier, complacent or seemingly indulgent, self-compassion motivates and results in you doing better work, leading to higher performance.[4]

Self-compassion versus self-criticism

Making personal changes can be daunting and intimidating: a self-compassionate perspective can make them less so. Even if you mess up, you've got your own back. Unlike self-esteem, which requires inflated self-evaluation, self-compassion protects against debilitating self-criticism. Or, as Lori Gottlieb writes in her riveting and hilarious book *Maybe You Should Talk to Someone*, self-compassion asks the question, *Am I human?* versus self-esteem, which asks, *Am I good or bad?* When people treat themselves with compassion, they are better able to honestly self-appraise, an important aspect of self-improvement and self-development. It allows for personal weaknesses to be identified, and rather than condemning the whole self you are motivated to improve these. Being self-compassionate is also a greater predictor of self-worth and lower narcissism than self-esteem – important ingredients in any relationship.[5]

A HEART-BREATHING MEDITATION TO EXPAND INNER COMPASSION

Your heart's energy centre is located in the middle of your chest. For a few moments, practise heart breathing.

1. Place a hand over your heart centre to help focus your attention. With each breath draw positive energy into your heart's centre as you inhale.

2. Hold your breath and feel your heart radiate a certain frequency of love. As you exhale, share this loving energy more deeply within.

3. With each breath, focus on this energy centre, breathing more deeply. Liberate any unwanted thoughts or energy from your body with each exhale. Continue breathing through the heart. Expand this love centre – your source of compassion, your self-compass.

A self-compassion growth mindset

One reason being more self-compassionate helps you recover better from setbacks or failures is because personal growth is possible with practice and effort. According to Stanford University psychology professor and author of *Mindset* Carol Dweck, this demonstrates an expansive or growth mindset – a view that character traits and abilities are malleable; the opposite of a fixed mindset where personality traits and abilities are believed to be set in stone. There's not much room for personal growth if you are of the opinion that who you are now will be the same in ten years' time.

A person displaying a growth mindset will keep trying to do better or be a better person after receiving negative feedback or having a negative encounter. And are, therefore, less likely to fall into a heap or descend the emotional spiral. On the other hand, if you believe abilities are fixed, making an effort is futile. When you drop judgement, it can be easier to confront negative aspects of yourself and strive to improve as you aren't as deterred by negative feedback. You can modify your behaviour with a sense of self-respect, kindness and compassion.

Self-compassion and authenticity

There's also a correlation between self-compassion and authenticity – founded on the notion your life does not have to be earnt; you are born worthy. Over the course of one week, participants of a University of Memphis study were asked to rate their levels of self-compassion ('Today, I showed caring, understanding and kindness towards myself') and authenticity ('Today, I felt authentic and genuine in my interactions with others'). On days participants reported being more compassionate towards themselves relative to their average level, they also reported greater feelings of authenticity.[6] When we're feeling authentic, being ourselves, we're not as concerned about social disapproval. We feel a sense of inner peace and joy – alignment. Neff describes this as 'wrapping one's pain in the warm embrace of self-compassion, positive feelings are generated that help balance the negative ones, allowing for more joyous states of mind'.[7] It's a positive way of relating to oneself that generates a sense of wellbeing. When we're internally content, not only do we feel more equilibrium, but others can sense it too.

People can sense authenticity as much as they can sense someone is being fake, and, as I have previously said, fake does not look good on anyone. When people feel authentic in their interactions with others, stronger relationships are forged. Whether that's feeling more satisfied in intimate relationships, or in compassionate workplaces that provide a respectful and supportive working environment. Studies have found that when leaders are seen as being true to themselves, an atmosphere of authenticity spreads throughout the workplace.[8] Even if we're put to the test and our sense of self is challenged or criticised, viewing ourselves as a work-in-progress helps authentically build our professional and personal identities.

MONITORING SELF-COMPASSION

Responses to these questions are a good measure of self-compassion. It's worth checking back every now and then to see how you're faring. Please rate yourself between one and five, where one is not at all and five is fully.

1. To what degree am I able to stop comparing myself to others?
   1 2 3 4 5

2. To what degree am I able to let go of the need to be perfect?
   1 2 3 4 5

3. To what degree am I able to treat and talk to myself kindly when going through a challenging time?
   1 2 3 4 5

4. To what degree do I believe I am enough?
   1 2 3 4 5

5. To what degree do I believe I am worthy?
   1 2 3 4 5

6. To what degree do I believe I am loveable?
   1 2 3 4 5

7. To what degree am I willing to embrace my whole self (warts and all)?
   1 2 3 4 5

For areas where you scored less than three, ask yourself: what can I do to raise my score? Take a moment to visualise and imagine how being more self-compassionate would feel, considering the flow-on effect to your relationships with others.

Mirror, mirror on the wall

Self-compassion is hard, even for 'experts' such as myself. I got so busy mothering everyone else, I forgot to mother myself. Not only did I lose my sense of humour, but the cacophony of other people's needs silenced my inner caregiver. All the wisdom I'd imbibed over the years, the books I'd read, presentations I'd listened to and given, and conferences I'd attended could not revive me.

It occurred to me, when it came to self-compassion I'd been sporting the cheap fake, not the real deal. I'd been extolling its virtues far and wide, believing I was taking care of my own needs, meditating for thirty minutes a day, ordering takeaway once a week, stopping to smell the roses. I had tricked myself into the illusion that I was looking after myself, all the while being a dutiful mother, daughter, sister, friend, partner, employee and civically minded citizen. Over the years, and with many competing demands for my attention, 'I' transitioned into 'i'. All this in the context of a pandemic, navigating working-from-home arrangements, writing this joyful book, the daily bombardment of gloomy global events, multiple lockdowns and the humdrum of domestic duties. To top it off, I was dealing with hot flushes and sleep deprivation courtesy of menopause (which I've since lovingly reframed as 'pausewoman'). Lockdown became my best friend. I went from social butterfly to foetal cocoon. Sick and tired of being sick and tired had become a tired excuse.

Then giving-itis engulfed me. I'd become such an expert in underplaying my physical and emotional health, I believed I could keep placing a plaster over a gaping wound. My first step towards activating a kinder, more compassionate self was turning towards others who could throw me a line. My doctor relayed that whatever she could provide in the way of additional medications or supplements would only form 30 per cent of my health picture. The remaining 70 per cent was up to me. After a lengthy consultation, her parting words hit me deeply: 'You know what you need to do', to which I thought, *No, I'm not sure I do*. Then as I walked towards the door, the clincher: 'Be kind to yourself.' Cue tears.

My inner compass was directionless – gone AWOL (absent without official ~~leave~~ love). Without a functional compass, my inner compassion whittled down to a non-functioning 'ion'. I needed to do something radical. I'd sacrificed myself far too long. There could be no shortcuts or quick fixes. It was time for me to invest in my heart's needs so I could return to the business of what I love doing – giving to others. This and this alone was the kindest thing I could do. The only thing. To fuel my depleted spirit; to summon bravery and heed my soul's call; to reconnect to nature, sunshine and my inner smile; to give back to myself, body, mind and spirit. I needed time and space to change my internal narrative to heal. A journey of self-discovery in Far North Queensland provided the seed. It was up to me to provide mental sunshine and water.

Once I embraced and acknowledged this, the wall of self-judgement collapsed. My entire being tilted back to smile mode. A quote in psychologist and meditation teacher Tara Brach's *Radical Compassion* book caught my attention. Zen teacher Charlotte Joko Beck said, 'Our incapacity to forgive is directly related to our ability to feel joy in our life.'[9] My path back to joy stemmed from wholeheartedly forgiving myself for any perceived wrongdoings. To move forward and disentangle myself from the past. Free myself of blame and give myself permission to release pain and trauma (self-inflicted and otherwise). To invite caring and kindness to my inner voice and commentary, embracing my self-compassion 'learner' status, even though I'd kidded myself I was advanced.

FEELING SELF-COMPASSION (NOT THINKING IT!)

Research shows supportive touch lowers cortisol levels and triggers neurotransmitters that boost wellbeing, including oxytocin and serotonin. If a friend or loved one isn't available, we can achieve a similar outcome ourselves.

1. Give yourself a hug, place your hand on your heart, or on an area of your body that's in pain, stroke your arms.

2. Hold any of these positions for a minimum of fifteen seconds and notice how that feels. Do you sense relief or release? If so, hold it a little longer and deepen and expand this sensation. Physically comforting your body increases feelings of love and tenderness.

3. Spend some time subtracting the thought process and soaking in the qualities of self-compassion – of love, kindness and acceptance.

My reason for sharing my ultimate self-compassion 'fail' is to help you understand personal growth is a journey. It's not enough to read the words and say, 'Job done.' Compassion – as with many of the topics in this book – is an inside job. It's as much about heart-set as it is mindset. No one can do self-compassion like you can. It needs to be given AIR (attention, intention and repetition). Otherwise, like so many of our resources, it remains dormant and silent.

To authentically become self-compassionate, we need to listen and honour our needs. To get to a place of acceptance not *exceptance*. While it may not require doing something as radical as my 'going troppo' sabbatical, repatterning a lifetime of inner talk, beliefs and modus operandi is a complex affair. We are constantly put to the test, whether it's relationship breakdowns, financial stress, health or grief – life is challenging enough with all the love and support in the world, but the love we most need is embodied within, when we are our own best friend and advocate.

No matter how important our loved ones are, there's no one more important than you. Do you hear me? I'll say it again in bold in case your eyes skipped a line.

No matter how important all our loved ones are, there's no one more important than you.

We all do foolish things from time to time, and nobody is perfect. So, you messed up here and there. You may feel a little fake or even a failure. Suppress your inner saboteur. Instead of feeling embarrassed or defensive, embrace your imperfections. It's time to relinquish the mask of imperfection, embracing a reframe of 'I'm perfection'. Please stop condemning *the whole* of you.

To be self-compassionate, first you must *become*. Bring to mind a true friend, mentor or even a higher being. What words would they offer you? Experiment in ways that feel well suited and authentic to you. Practise, and practise some more, until you might wobble but you don't topple.

In time, just like me, you'll notice you're smiling more, feeling more inwardly joyful and content. You'll be able to smile and laugh at your imperfections and be more lighthearted about your self-perceived flaws. Self-compassion with a smile offers a powerful opportunity to replace inner judgement with inner joy, inner loathing with inner loving, and inner grief with inner gratitude. Embedding the Laughter Effect into self-compassion rituals is a heart-set we can all aspire to. It's one that welcomes and expands upon love in all forms. Nurturing inner-compassion is one of the kindest practices you can bestow upon yourself – because, as we've established, the gorgeous you, warts and all, matters. As motivational author, the late Louise Hay, inspired, 'You've been criticising yourself for years and it hasn't worked. Try approving of yourself and see what happens.'

10

Joyful Journaling and Positive Reframing

*I can shake off everything as I write; my sorrows disappear
and my courage is reborn*

—Anne Frank

Turning to the written word to relieve one's stress or narrate one's story is a strong tool to process challenging emotions and journey into our innermost thoughts. A refuge for negative waste. But what of its potential to foster positive emotion and enhance the good in your life? The Laughter Effect adds another element to journaling's therapeutic capacity, expanding on positive emotion in an authentic and natural way and directing the patterning of our inner mind to an inspired, more joyful version of our self. While our thoughts are generated by the mind, joyful journaling also creates harmony between mind and body, and boosts mental health and wellbeing. It's important at any time – especially when life gets messy.

Joyful journaling is different from writing a diary. It integrates the Laughter Effect into the written word, providing another means to strengthen neural pathways towards humour, laughter and levity. It is an intentional way of writing to enhance positive personal growth and psychological resilience. It's not about denying the exploration of adverse events or being superficially chirpy like so much on social media; it's about doing our darndest to deny negative emotions taking up permanent residency. Or, as the saying goes, 'Your issues become your tissues.'

It doesn't require a radical shift where there's no place for negative thoughts, but rather it's a gentle nudge towards the more subtle, beneficial ones. It's also a technique that captures and intensifies fleeting positive emotions. Joyful journaling hones our ability to seek and expand upon the light in a situation, no matter how infinitesimal that might be. Once the door towards levity has been opened, you can question your mind's messaging and choose whether or not to believe what it thinks. In doing so, it launches you on a path of self-discovery to expand and develop qualities that serve you well.

Body and mind serve as a depository of emotion and memory. Unfurling our innermost thoughts into language can improve our mental state. In writing about a stressful event, your body will respond in kind. It will tense – teeth and jaw clenching, heart racing and your breath held. Recounting life's pleasures, or the things that are going well in our day, encourages a sense of peace and calm. We exhale, sigh, unclench, untense, and even smile. That's the Laughter Effect.

Take a moment here to ask yourself (in your head or writing it down), *Am I feeling any stress in my body right now? If so, where is it stored and what can I do to release it?* Sometimes awareness is all it takes to dissolve emotional stickiness.

Now ask yourself, *Where do I feel joy and how can I feel more of it?* In this case, you're inviting an opportunity to bring your emotions to the forefront. As your body cannot think, you're giving it a chance to express itself in its own language. As previously discussed, the longer emotions hang around, the more they influence physiology – in both a good and not-so-good way.

A mix of contrasting emotions plays out for our attention. This is explained in the following enchanting fable, 'The Tale of Two Wolves'. In teaching his grandson about life, an old man says to the boy:

'A fight is going on inside me. It is a terrible fight, and it is between two wolves. One is evil – he is anger, envy, sorrow, regret, greed, arrogance, self-pity, guilt, resentment, inferiority, lies, false pride, superiority, and ego.'

'The other is good – he is joy, peace, love, hope, serenity, humility, kindness, benevolence, empathy, generosity, truth, compassion, and faith. The same fight is going on inside you – and inside every other person, too.'

The grandson thinks about it for a minute and then asks his grandfather, 'Which wolf will win?'

The old man simply replies, 'The one you feed.'

Which wolf are you feeding? Negative thinking is normal, yet it can become greedy for our attention, unfavourably impacting on our mental health and mood, sapping energy. As we've explored, our thoughts can be our own worst enemy, sending us spiralling emotionally to a place where our inadequacies breed. Negative emotions narrow attention, cognition and physiology towards coping with an immediate threat or problem.[1] They can be overwhelming, which is why we're drawn to write about the challenging stuff, to make sense of our struggles.

Joyful journaling reveals a side that for many is buried deep in dust and cobwebs. So much so, you may question it ever existed. A challenge we face is the transitory nature of positive thoughts. They're a whisper, rather than a holler, and create a misperception that they are unimportant. We rarely notice them unless they are obvious celebratory days – perhaps a birthday, promotion or wedding anniversary. That's why we need to pay more attention to them. Journaling with positive intent is an effective way of taming negative thinking.

We can feed our inner wolf of goodness to build our store of positive emotions, broadening and building lasting social, psychological and practical resources that help us deal with a wide range of life's challenges and tune into multiple intelligences – physical, intellectual, emotional and spiritual. That's not to say there isn't merit in dumping one's woes, but without bringing in an opportunity for lightness, like bullies, they'll knock us to the ground.

FEEDING THE BIG BAD WOLF

→ Describe an instance when you fought off possibilities for positive transformation.

→ Were your actions motivated by fear, anger or disappointment?

→ Thinking about this instance now, is there any lingering resistance to positive transformation? If so, create a plan to help work through it.

→ Is there something else you're currently resisting? How would your story change if you surrendered to resistance?

→ In your life in general, how much does FEAR (false evidence appearing real) hold you back? From your passions, from relationships, from being authentic and truthful – AKA the real and beautiful you?

The objective distance that is created when we reflect on our circumstances enables us to challenge our story. How true or untrue, negative or positive. In *Writing to Awaken: A Journey of Truth, Transformation and Self-Discovery*, Mark Matousek describes how we become the 'Witness' in the journaling process. It's a mindful lens on a new realm of possibilities and perspectives, connecting us to the right hemisphere of the brain associated with feelings, intuition and emotional intelligence. It's a way of giving ourselves advice. By cultivating the Witness, we realise we are the storytellers, not the stories. Journaling paves the way for new insights of self-understanding – to those *aha* and *ha, ha* moments that unlock hidden aspects of consciousness. It's an invaluable resource, as Albert

Einstein observed, 'No problem can be solved from the same level of consciousness that created it.'

Matousek also advocates embracing a Beginner's Mind, pure and innocent, to meet each moment without prejudice. It allows for many possibilities, helping to reveal that much of your life plays out unnoticed, or is taken for granted, whereas an expert's mind can be blind, closed to new perspectives or possibilities, tarnished by judgement or cynicism. It means we can embrace thoughts, beliefs and feelings that haven't naturally been in our frame of consciousness with curiosity – and even excitement. Just as a child might enthuse over their first journey on a train, the written word enables us to train our mind from one track to one of diversity.

Negative thoughts won't disappear, but in time and with practice, they can become less dominant – the revelation of an upside of a downside. For example, giving a voice to anger may release repressed emotions or reveal its root cause. Consider a tiny match. When struck, it can illuminate a darkened room. The same applies to our thoughts. As it is physically impossible to simultaneously inhabit conflicting mindsets, you can consciously and intentionally change your tune. As Megan Hayes describes in *Write Yourself Happy: The Art of Positive Journalling*, 'feeling positive is never mandatory but it is a possibility'. Writing in the key of positivity is a choice we can all make.

. . . .

Viktor Frankl, author of *Man's Search for Meaning*, wisely shared that when you choose your attitude, you cannot be a victim. Victimhood is a cruel and greedy master. Too often we're blinded by its grip. My bowel cancer diagnosis could have been a sentence to victimhood. Emotionally overwrought, I was saved by the written word when I heeded my soul's voice to reach for pen and paper as a means of regaining some control. Early in my journaling practice, I realised how my thoughts impacted my feelings, and how much control I had. If I focused on those 'f' words – fear, fed-up and frustration – that's how I felt: fearful and frustrated. On the other hand, if I considered something remotely positive – even only for one moment – that's where my thoughts and emotions went.

From this vantage point, I could choose to remain in a more uplifting space or succumb to negative feelings of helplessness or hopelessness. With positive intention and attention, new insights would come to mind, highlighting beliefs, feelings and thoughts that were not serving me well. Once brought to the light, I could challenge and change them – or not. The choice was mine, and mine alone. In the silence of introspection, a private channel unlocked to my intuitive, wiser self. Here was a sacred space in which I could intentionally invite greater inquiry into my practice. It was my first experience writing with the Laughter Effect rather than leaving uplifting emotions to chance. It helped free me from my negative 'comfort' zone. The words may have formed in my head, but with practice and focus they also penetrated my body and soul.

The more we hone our inner voice to listen, the more we hear

We gain the most when we welcome a sense of kindness, acceptance and even laughter into our written exploration of whatever's going on in our life. Writing from the heart, through a laughter lens, allows us to first reveal, and then embrace the vast dimension of self with humility and even possibly humour, allowing us time to play with our mind. It enables us to consider aspects we rarely pay attention to – our gifts, strengths, and all the people in our life and experiences that have made us who we are. It helps us to focus on our body, physically and emotionally conditioned by the past, over many, many years, and also gives us space to reflect on the excuses we come up with for not doing what we want to do, preventing us from living our bravest most joy- and passion-filled life, or to where

SEROTONIN SISTER

I'm not much of a writer, something that was reinforced by my high school English teacher. I'm not sure if journaling's for me and doubt it will come easily.

It's amazing how some things we're told stay with us for years while others pass in one ear and out the other. Thankfully, there's no risk of your journaling being graded. Besides, we don't have to believe what others say about ourselves, and if you are prone to doing so, I suggest focusing on the good that's said. Journaling is a means of transferring thoughts from both your conscious and unconscious mind onto paper – the fun ones and also the messy ones. No matter how finessed the language, the writing process creates a little distance, enabling you to challenge and release unhelpful thought patterns. Make a start and see what unfolds. You really can't go wrong. A great place to begin your journaling practice may be challenging beliefs around what your English teacher said!

our personal roadblocks lie. Our pen on paper or finger on keyboard becomes our baton – determining how we choose to conduct our life.

SUPERPOWERS, ACTIVATE! TIME TO DREAM BIG

→ What's your superpower – otherwise known as your strengths and gifts?

→ What superpower do you wish you had? Why would you like this power and how would you put it to use?

→ In what ways would activating this superpower on a regular basis make you stronger and more connected to your life's meaning and purpose?

Energy flows where attention goes – reframing with the Laughter Effect

Megan Hayes says, 'Writing positively is not necessarily about wearing rose-tinted glasses, it can be like taking dirty glasses off.' A critical aspect of journaling with the Laughter Effect is reframing stressful or painful situations. When traumatic or stressful events are reframed with a laughter mindset, the brain recalls these events in a different light, lessening associated trauma. It demonstrates another way of thinking, where problems can be reframed as opportunities for learning and new perspectives can be gleaned. It also remedies against 'shoulds' – I should feel this way, or I shouldn't be feeling that way. This has a flow-on effect into our body and our immunity to stress. Reframing with levity or finding the funniness in a stressful situation develops personal resilience and mental freedom. It has not only been one of the most impactful practices I have introduced in my life, but also – as reported to me – in my clients' lives.

One of the biggest reframes I achieved in my life was to do with the word 'cancer'– from a big 'C' to a little 'c', acknowledging that the cancer was residing in one small area of my rectum. The rest of me (at the time, I had my fingers crossed) was healthy and well. Lessening my emotional load created more space for healing and wellbeing. It also helped my children cope through this process: as long as Mum did not have the big 'C', there was considerably more hope. Our collective future brightened. We could all deal better with the little 'c'.

Later, ahead of my bowel reversal operation (which, to me, implied a change in direction – backwards), I reframed the terminology to a 'bowel reconnection'. Some may say this is purely semantics, but, for me, this reframe was significant. It was my language infused with positivity. I wanted to be reconnected to newness and future possibilities where my bowel would be bound together for the journey ahead, not tied to what had been. I even changed my work computer password to Reconnected@120 (referring to a Jewish tradition of blessing someone to live to 120 in health and happiness). This action alleviated much anxiety going into that operation and helped me regain some control over an overwhelming feeling of helplessness being at the mercy of the surgeon's blade, yet again.

Reframing in the key of gratitude made me realise that no matter what was going on in my external environment, I could always question and change my internal environment by intentionally calling on the Laughter Effect. Challenging my narrative, I gleaned valuable insights. In time, being able to view this as a trauma happening *for* me, not *to* me. That's the transformative aspect. A wise philosopher of our times, Homer (Simpson, of course) described this as a 'crisitunity' – the opportunity within a crisis. The gift is unlikely to occur while the trauma is unfolding – generally only after the worst of it has passed. To some it can manifest as an epiphany; to others it's a sense of knowingness, from *aha* moments to *ha, ha* moments, with the Laughter Effect, and vice versa. No matter how it's discovered, therein lies an opportunity for healing. Taking your life in a new direction and helping to counter victimhood.

CASE STUDY: Rewriting your story

A client, 'Susan', had a perfect life on paper: long-term content marriage, successful career, children and more recently grandchildren, with finances to indulge life's luxuries. She wasn't joyless, but she was far from joyful. Perhaps she felt joy was not in her remit. That happiness had to be earnt rather than being a right. Aside from introducing her to gratitude practices, mindful breathing and individual endorphin triggers, I noted her creative flair and suggested positive journaling. To write in the key of joy: mapping it out across her life, exploring when she felt most and least connected to it, who she was with, what she was doing and, most importantly, sensing how joy felt in her body?

In our next session, Susan eagerly shared an 'aha' moment: a realisation that she had earnt the 'bad girl' label when she was young. Competing for attention with three other siblings close in age, Susan acted out as her way in. All these years, she had carried the torch of unworthiness: a 'bad girl' doesn't deserve to be happy. Journaling with the Laughter Effect allowed the light of insight in. It released the stagnant, dense energy of how she was defined in the past, to a place she could safely confront her inner saboteurs. Reframing her past from 'bad girl' to 'a girl wanting loving and deserved attention' paved the way for a more joyful and optimistic future. Over the weeks, I was struck by her visible transformation, mirroring her lighter mind. Her capacity to accept joy as a right manifested stronger with each session.

Simply recounting traumatic events isn't sufficient to shift stubborn pain. It takes courage and introspection, together with practice and effort, to positively rewire the brain. Repetitive action. Even the smallest opening towards lightness creates a shift in perspective. In time, neural pathways to positivity and joy become strengthened, flowing to our emotional, spiritual and physical body.

REFRAMING YOUR PAIN

When going through a tough or painful time it's easy to get stuck in the moment, not being able to view the situation in a more expansive light. On paper, bring to mind a time or event in your life that was somewhat stressful, painful or challenging. It's best to begin by choosing something not overwhelmingly painful or challenging.

1. As you reflect back to this event, compile a list of as many positives as you can. What can you be grateful for? Keep in mind gratitude can be past-, present- or even future-focused. Can you identify any opportunities for growth or learning?

2. Now that some time has passed, is it possible to find any lightness, even funniness?

3. Rewrite this episode acknowledging some of the positives you highlighted. Doing so will help your brain recall this event with a little less trauma, lessening associated emotional pain.

CASE STUDY: Reframing and journaling

One of my clients, 'Ben', a marketing executive in his early thirties, hit a low when the love of his life became the love of another's. Heartbroken and humourless, he turned to me to help raise his spirits. Initially he was so scarred by the breakup that he struggled to find any resultant positives. Yet over the course of a few weeks, positive reframing and joyful journaling expanded and widened his perspective, elevating his mood and mindset.

At the beginning of our sessions, I explained that it wasn't about denying the tough stuff – how hurt he felt or how much he missed his ex – rather, it was about acknowledging how much power Ben held over his emotional state. If he chose to dwell only on the souring of the relationship, that's all he would see. With some gentle guidance he began shifting from a viewpoint of this being the end of the world to the end of one chapter. Through journaling with positive intent, Ben began to see the many opportunities that arose from one door closing, and rather than passively waiting for another to open, he gave himself permission to push a new door open. To meet new people, have gratitude for the time spent with his former partner and the moments of joy they shared, and to reflect on what he'd gained and learnt from the relationship – such as identifying a need to nurture emotional intelligence. Thinking about that allowed him to raise a smile. I even suggested he write (and not necessarily send, unless he especially wanted to) a letter to his ex, thanking him for all the good times they shared.

When reframed as a potential for growth and an opportunity for a fresh start, both his future and past looked less bleak. Rather than feel like a failure, which is how he initially presented, the written word empowered a belief in himself as someone who was loveable and brave enough to risk taking a chance on love. Within weeks, he developed inner resources making him more resilient and prepared for any downturn in life events – not solely relationship breakdowns. Supportive joy-sparking mindfulness practices subtly transformed his tears of sadness to tears of joy. It's not to say his heart didn't ache, but applying the principles of the Laughter Effect to his breakup pieced him back together to a more optimistic, lighter and stronger version of himself.

Why feed the inner wolf of negativity when you can feed its adversary?

Inviting questions into your practice focusing on gratitude, hope, curiosity, serenity, love, awe and joy will keep the growling wolf at bay. I acknowledge that writing may not come easily or naturally for some.

Despite what you may have been told in school, there are no right and wrongs: just write. You'll find your voice. You'll find your way. Whether prose, random thoughts, stream of consciousness writing or a marksman's favourite – bullet points. Whether you do it as the first thing in your day or the last, it doesn't matter. Although, a bonus of journaling with the Laughter Effect before bed is that it will positively orient your mind, feeding your subconscious and enriching your dreams.

If you journal electronically, despite what autocorrect may dictate, there's no need to pay too much attention to grammar or spelling. It's more important to fully explore and express your desires and allow whatever bubbles to the surface to breathe.

Adding mindful pauses catches ourselves in the act of thinking, reclaiming control over our mind's in-built negativity bias. It provides an opportunity to ask yourself, *Are these thoughts, beliefs or emotions helping or hindering?* A process further enhanced by tuning into bodily sensations as you write – your breath (whether you're holding it), heart rate or sensations in the gut, throat or chest directs our attention to the charge of our inner voice.

Please be patient and kind to yourself in the process. That can mean one word at a time and not pressuring yourself by indulging your inner judgement or criticism that you 'aren't doing it right'. If you're feeling internal resistance, try *journaling light*. Create affirmations. *I am loving journaling with the Laughter Effect* can be a good one to whet your journaling appetite. Affirmations can motivate you towards attaining your goals. To be your personal cheerleader. When we repeat these words regularly, outwardly or silently, our brain begins to take their word for it.

This new truth becomes hardwired in your brain. A bit like manifesting but with a lot more mastery.

If the suggestion to positively engineer your written word is a little daunting, perhaps reframe this process as scripted daydreaming. A space where you can dwell in the playground of your mind. Or derive inspiration from leading teachers in this space. Julia Cameron – artist, poet, playwright, novelist, filmmaker and author of *The Artist's Way* – advocates for a Morning Pages practice: three pages of long-form, stream-of-consciousness writing, done first thing in the morning. It's about anything and everything that crosses your mind. It's a great way to develop clarity and set the tone for the day ahead, dumping any unwanted thoughts on the page. A fertile space for 'aha' moments that have transformed countless lives around the globe – mine included.

Although, as we've discussed, free-flow writing is different from joyful journaling, which does not leave creating an upbeat inner environment to chance. Traditional journaling also comes with a risk of wallowing in negativity rather than rousing yourself from the swamp of your mind. Churning through the mud of adversity takes its toll. It can leave a pungent aroma that trails through your day. Joyful journaling is a potent reminder that no single story, no matter how substantial, can fully define you, as you always have the power to change. Just as my client Susan did. The process allows the mud in our mind to settle and clarity to rise to the surface. On the written page, grief can be transformed into gratitude, fear into love, weakness into strength, inner judgement to inner knowledge, grudge into grace, darkness to light, and limited beliefs to endless possibilities. Our mindset is an inside job, as is our happiness, as playwright, screenwriter and author Catherine Ann Jones penned in *Heal Yourself with Writing*: 'Use happy memories to water the small seed of becoming whole.'

With practice you'll begin feeling a difference in your bones – particularly your funny bone. A hint of positivity. A jot of joy. Regaining mastery of your life – an essential attribute of wellbeing.

As word artisans, we can craft our own inspiring story. To say yes to our deepest hopes and desires. Make the sweetest of dreams our reality. When perception of our story changes, so too does our world. As English romantic poet William Wordsworth wrote, 'Fill your paper with the breathings of your heart.' That's when the real magic begins, towards infinite potential. When you're the 'pilot of your soul' (thanks Elton John!) the blue sky is the limit. Which wolf will you feed? *Remember, you always have a choice.* Journaling with the Laughter Effect mines the gold from the silt. Change your story. Change your life.

Journaling activities

The following activities will help you get started on your new diet. A diet of positivity.

Some ground rules:

- Please don't overcomplicate things. There's no need to purchase the 'perfect' journal in order to begin. Keep in mind, there's no right. Just write!

- Create mindful moments for positivity. Focus on what's going well in your day and grow that goodness.

- Engage your Beginner's Mind and become a Witness to your thoughts and emotions. A practice can be something as simple as crafting an affirmation.

- If you're undergoing an especially challenging moment, let your journaling skip ahead into the future. To a scenario created in your mind's eye that's full of hope, and an expressed desire for easier and more joyful times ahead.

A focus on self-compassion

Journaling can help tone your self-compassion muscle. Here are a few prompts to get you going.

- When you fail or make a mistake, what are some of the thoughts that run through your mind?

- How critical or otherwise is your inner voice? What is it telling you? *Toughen up, Stop complaining,* or *You've got this!*

- What would you say to a friend or loved one in this exact situation?

- Do you acknowledge shortcomings and failure as experiences shared by everyone?

- Do you keep your negative feelings in perspective?

- Write down the many ways you are compassionate and kind to your friends or loved ones.

Acknowledge ALL feelings. Even the uncomfortable ones. Embracing and accepting all parts of yourself and your full range of human emotions is key to healing. Journaling can highlight that feelings come and go. They do not define you.

Growing gratitude

- Write about a life event in the key of gratitude.

- What aspects of yourself are you grateful for? Expand on what others might be grateful for in you.

Jottings on joy

- Who or what in your life brings you the most joy and how can you get more of it?

- When you're focusing on these things, how does it make you feel – mentally, emotionally and physically?

Leaning towards love

- Where do you feel love in your body? Let the written word guide and deepen your embodied experience of love.

- What steps can you take to grow your capacity to love and be loved?

Flow baby flow

- Describe an experience of flow in your life when you were completely immersed in an activity and time seemed to stop. How can you access this state more often?

Curating curiosity

- What piques your curiosity? What fascinates you?

- What would you like to learn more about?

Awesome awe

- Bring to mind a moment you felt really connected to awe. A sunset, magical encounter or oneness with a higher force.

Serenity now

- Write down what you need to feel more serenity in your life. Express that need compassionately and without judgement. Make a plan and identify the necessary steps to move towards it.

Power up passion

- What's your earliest memory of an activity you were passionate about? How did it make you feel? Where in your body do you feel this passion? Have you continued to engage in this activity? Why or why not?

- What might your life look and feel like if you started saying *yes* to the things that fill your heart with passion? Be specific.

Find the funniness

- Relive a fun or funny experience. Feel free to recall an event from childhood. Include as much detail as you can. Allow this feeling to expand until you're smiling or laughing along with the memory.

- Explore and outline how you can fire up more fun and funniness in your life.

11

The Last Laugh

Life is brighter on the laughter-side
—Ros Ben-Moshe

It's been a joy and privilege journeying with you through the Laughter Effect. My wish is that these varied techniques and practices will enrich and enliven not only your life but also the lives around you. With intention, attention and practice, you can cultivate a more positive and optimistic internal environment, hardwiring uplifting emotions. This body-mind practice expands and builds personal resources to buoy your spirits, even during life's prickly moments.

The more the Laughter Effect forms a beat in your day, the greater its ability to joy-start communication, connection and performance – at home, work, anywhere. With repetition, your mind will be equipped to drop into the elevating energy of the Laughter Effect more readily – to catalyse positive energy into motion, no matter how big or small. To live it.

You may face hurdles along the way. With the dominance of technology in so many aspects of our lives, there is an increased need for these techniques in order to reconnect us to the qualities that make us human. When it comes to humorous or playful exchanges, we need to be mindful of the all-important social dimension. If the messenger is a screen rather than a full-mouthed grin IRL (in real life), the Laughter Effect lessens, and our brain's applause is curtailed. LOL and ROFL are poor cousins to real life gut-aching rolling on the floor laughter. But it doesn't mean technology can't be used to our advantage. Being able to see someone's face, even if they're on the other side of the world, switches on mirror neurons, and when matched with a smile or laughter, it signals our DOSE of wellbeing. And of course, there's more potential for the conversational punctuation effect of laughter to kick in.

There's no need to feel overwhelmed or daunted by the idea of putting the Laughter Effect into practice. For optimal results, make it your own by choosing how you'd like to weave it into your life. If at the end of the day you don't feel like joyful journaling, you could watch a comedy. If you're not in the mood for a smile meditation, instead listen to an affirmative podcast. Or if you don't want to commit to an entire Laughter Yoga session, choose to power laugh for ten seconds. In the following final chapter, you will find a selection of practices and techniques to help make parenting more fulfilling and enjoyable, relationships more fun and rewarding, illness or adversity more manageable, workplaces happier spaces and life more loveable.

Leaning into the Laughter Effect may not conquer the world's ills, but it will align it closer to love, and ripple out into the broader community. As we've explored, it's both a heart-set and mindset providing moments for positive transformation and healing – body, mind and soul. A strategy to transform *ooh* and *aah* moments to *aha* and *ha, ha*. It's too important to leave to chance. Timetable laughter. Timetable joy. Be loving, appreciative and kind to yourself – always. Please don't keep these learnings to yourself. The world is a smaller and more loving place when people are bound by laughter. Share the ~~love~~ laugh. As one of the wisest doctors of all times, Dr Seuss, pronounced, 'You have brains in your head. You have feet in your shoes. You can steer yourself any direction you choose.' Choose the Laughter Effect.

In gratitude and appreciation for your time. Wishing you much love, laughter, joy and happiness.

Ros ☺

The Laughter Effect in Practice

As you're now familiar with the theory and practice of the Laughter Effect, it's time to make a plan – to identify aspects of your life that the Laughter Effect will best support and enrich. It's fine to start slowly, though the most benefit to your overall wellbeing will be attained if you select at least one of these to integrate into your home and/or work daily. Dip into whichever techniques and practices speak to you. Sense the inner call of your physical, social, emotional, mental and spiritual needs. Be mindful that each day has a different tone.

Parenting with the Laughter Effect

Here are some simple and fun tips and activities to brighten your day. They will assist in building loving and joyful familial connections and allow you to better manage the inevitable stresses of parenting. Over time, the Laughter Effect will become fully integrated into your parenting style, making for happier 'big kids' and little kids.

- **Build your humour capacity.** Find and share funniness at mealtimes with household members about things you saw or heard during your day. (For more ideas, please refer to chapter five, Our Sixth Sense – Humour.)

- **Get physical.** Physical comedy (funny facial gestures, unusual physical movements – the 'funny walk' for one) works wonders with the littlies. As your children get older, introduce verbal humour and opportunities to be playfully inventive and creative.

- **Create a comedy/sitcom-viewing ritual.** *Sunday night silly*, or *Friday night funny*. Watch together, bundled on the couch.

- **Avoid creating drama kings and queens and create comedians.** A child's response is in part influenced by a parent's, which is why responding to minor mishaps with humour lessens drama. For example, find the humour in a tumble or fall. 'Did that tree trip you up? What a naughty tree!' Ha ha ha.

- **Maintain perspective.** Just like so many childhood phases, toilet humour is just that – a phase.

- **Make a game plan.** Whether it's something spontaneous like hide-and-seek or a formal board game like *Apples to Apples* – one of our favourites. Choose something that will garner giggles and not become overly serious or competitive!

- **Create family in-jokes or fun, loving nicknames.** I'd probably get into trouble if I divulged ours, but over the years we've harvested a wide array of nicknames.

- **Make someone's quirky trait a treat.** *Laughingly* and lovingly jesting about someone's idiosyncrasy, in a way that demonstrates they're perfectly imperfect, imparts an important resilience tool.

- **Don't take yourself too seriously.** Occasionally make funny blunders to give your child a chuckle. This shows it's okay to have fun and be a bit silly.

- **Organise a scavenger hunt with smiley-face badges or stickers.** Everyone's a winner in a smiley scavenger hunt. Encourage everyone to wear as much of the bounty as they can.

- **Praise and reward good behaviour and other accomplishments with loving smiles.** Never pass up an opportunity to acknowledge and speak up the good in your child, or your partner.

- **Create opportunities to have fun and laugh together.** What does this mean for your family? Picnics, themed dinners, excursions or holidays – whatever nurtures quality bonding.

- **First thing in the morning, place a smile on your dial.** Share widely with your loved ones, especially the grumpy ones! (If you need a refresher, please refer to chapter seven about smiling.)

- **Improvise funny bedtime stories and invite your child to contribute.** This can be such a fun ritual, especially if they include sound effects.

- **Adopt a fur baby.** A puppy or kitten will do wonders to bring out your family's inner child and playful side. We welcomed a chocolate-brown labrador pup into our family at the beginning of the pandemic and named her LOLA: not after the legendary Kinks song, but an acronym for Laugh Out Loud Always. Her playful and loving antics made lockdown days brighter and brought our family unit closer.

- **Practise gratitude.** Create a gratitude jar and contribute notes of appreciation and gratitude you have received or observed. On a weekly basis dig in and share with one another. (See chapter eight, Gleeful Gratitude, for more tips on growing goodness.)

- **Reward kindness.** Compliment your child's actions when they've prioritised another person's needs or given of themselves generously.

The Laughter Effect for relationships

Make laugh, not war. As previously discussed, a good sense of humour consistently tops the 'must have' list in a partner. As life unfolds, this can seem more like an unattainable wish, as shared laugh-out-loud moments might wane as stress and life's obstacles get in the way. The Laughter Effect helps remind us of what's important and why we fell in love with our partner in the first instance. It's a potent way to maintain equilibrium, lessen stress and keep the relationship spark glowing.

- **Make smiling eye contact.** The pulse of our day is largely set the moment we first open our eyes and breathe in the energy of a new day. Set your dial to smile and encourage behaviour you'd like to receive in turn from your partner. (You'll recall reading about mirror neurons in chapter seven.)

- **Schedule time for a shared laugh.** Select a sitcom you both love chuckling through, listen to a funny podcast or go to a comedy show.

- **Share humour.** If something funny happened in your day, don't keep it to yourself – magnify its potency and share it.

- **Be present with each other.** Avoid staring at your phones when you could be enjoying each other's company. There's a greater likelihood for moments of amusement when you live in the now together.

- **Spend time with friends or family who make you feel good and bring out your laughter.** Perhaps this isn't possible all the time, but when there's a choice, seize it.

- **Smile mirror.** Sit opposite one another, stare the other in the face and see who can last the longest before smiling. Be prepared for the smiles to burst into laughter.

- **Wherever possible, avoid going to bed angry with one another.** Try to find humour in a stressful situation to defuse animosity. Or even say something like, 'I'm sure we'll find this funny when we reflect back on this in the future.' These strategies act as circuit breakers, paving the way for better communication. While at times it can be challenging, this is a *laughskill* worth persevering with and practising.

- **Be playful.** As we know, this may not necessarily result in laughter but will connect to shared joy and the lighter side of life.

- **Create in-jokes that only you know about.** Not sure if I should admit this, but Danny and I have a funny habit of classifying people as animals they resemble. We'll giggle about a catch up with 'the retriever', 'the beaver', 'the albatross' or 'the giraffe'.

- **Praise your partner when they activate the Laughter Effect.** When you grow these skills together, their impact can be far greater – individually and as a couple.

- **Be kind to one another.** Authentic and generous acts of kindness spark inner or outer smiles. Make the many micro-moments of the day count. Offer to make your partner a cup of tea or coffee, or share household chores.

- **Relive the fun.** As far as your mind is concerned, reminiscing is almost as good as the real thing. Look through old photos. Even make a date to revisit the places where the laughter happened.

- **Give each other endearing and fun pet names.** It's amazing how enduring pet names can be. One of ours derived from the name of an oversized bear we were gifted BC (before children).

- **Be game.** Dedicate an evening to play – trivia games, Scrabble, Bananagrams, Rummikub – whatever you both find fun and entertaining. Where there's play, laughter's not far behind.

- **Grow gratitude.** Make a ritual of sharing three things that went well in your day, or acts or attributes you're grateful for in your partner.

- **Find a way to bring more laughter into a bland day.** Be spontaneous and improvise. Catch your partner by the element of surprise. Transform your kitchen into a dance studio – turn up the music, raid the utensils drawers for drumstick equivalents and sing and dance like there's no tomorrow.

- **Lessen 'toothpaste tube moments'.** A phenomenon where how a partner squeezes the toothpaste tube, and whether or not the tube's cap is replaced, can prime arguments, expanding to broader relationship criticism. Regularly activating the Laughter Effect helps lessen irritation and frustration about the little things. Remember the red Mazda (p.148). Whatever you focus on, that's what grows; it's up to you. 'Toothpaste tube moments' or toothy smiling ones.

Activating the laughter effect during illness or adversity

Even during illness or adversity, amplifying positive qualities will make you feel better. Activating a laughter mindset optimises healing potential. Anchoring in the uplifting energy of the Laughter Effect primes body, mind and spirit towards wellness and away from illness. It accentuates the light – supporting you through this challenging time.

- **Begin positive journaling.** Use this as an opportunity to highlight what is going well in your day – the parts of your body that are functioning well, your support circle, aspects of your environment you appreciate, micro-moments of contentedness. Write in the key of positivity, looking for and expanding the light, no matter how seemingly trivial. (Refer to chapter ten for positive journaling tips.)

- **Reframe challenges in an empowering language.** Adopt a language of positivity and hope. Challenge your story and rewrite it in a fresh and empowering light. Doing so will lighten your load by lessening associated trauma. (Refer to chapter ten for more tips on reframing.)

- **Smile – to others and yourself.** This cues the endorphin flow, your body's pain management system, enhancing feelings of wellbeing and diminishing pain. Create a smile schedule, regularly placing a heartfelt smile on your face long enough to feel its embrace. Embed smiling into your daily meditation practice or deepen your inner and outer smile with a focused smiling meditation. (Refer to the smiling meditation in chapter seven.)

- **Surround yourself with people who lift your spirits.** This can be easier said than done, but where possible, spend time with people who make you feel more optimistic about your situation. Those friends or family members you can have a 'normal' conversation with – to let loose and have a laugh. Where you can forget about your issues for a while and just be you, free of an attachment to your present predicament.

- **Gift yourself a power laugh.** Power laughing for the health of it for ten seconds will do wonders to shift feelings of frustration, fear or anxiety. Aim to build up to one minute. Set your timer and laugh! For a practice that incorporates deep breathing, try laughter intervals. (Refer to chapter three.)

- **Be kind to yourself and soothe yourself with self-compassion.** Place a hand on your heart, offer words of loving support and encouragement, or smile wholeheartedly within. If you struggle with this, consider what you might say to a loved one going through something similar and then offer these sentiments to yourself.

- **Breathe.** Each day, check in with your breath. How shallow, deep, fast or slow is it? Spend a few moments optimising oxygen exchange, exhaling slightly longer than your inhalation. For example, breathe in for a count of three, and exhale for a count of four. After a few breath cycle repetitions the relaxation response will kick in, signalling your parasympathetic nervous system to bring calm and peace. Focus your attention on breathing in and out of your heart centre. Feel your breath enter this sacred space and feel it leave. With each breath expand the energy around your heart space. Notice how your mind and body respond, as you sink into the calm. You can also add positive intent into your practice: breathing in newness, healing and joy; exhaling negativity, stress or disease.

- **Count your blessings.** Notice, pause and absorb the good in your day. Each day, bring to mind or write at least three things you're grateful for. You can also be future grateful for an outcome you'd like to happen. Embody and extend the quality of thankfulness in the present moment. The more you seek, the more you will see. (Refer to the gratitude practices in chapter eight.)

- **Find the funny.** When facing adversity, a common fallout is the loss of our sense of humour. If you can't find anything funny about your current situation, look outside of it. Turn to the internet or social media for inspiration, or a favourite comedian who will brighten your spirits no matter what.

- **Laugh out loud.** Join a Laughter Yoga club (online or in person), choose comedies or light-hearted viewing or podcasts. Laugh free of judgement (self or other) – at yourself in the mirror, or when you're in the shower or in the car. (Refer to other intentional laughter exercises in chapter three.)

- **Drop the guilt.** Include as many things as possible on a regular basis that bring you joy and make you feel better about yourself. Have a massage, watch a cherished movie, indulge in your favourite food or tune into an uplifting podcast. Whatever feeds your soul.

- **Conduct a gratitude body scan.** Spend time sensing into your body and giving thanks for all the hard work it does day in, day out without being asked. (Refer to chapter eight.)

For further exploration on how to create a laughter mindset during illness or adversity, you may benefit from my memoir and healing guide, *Laughing at cancer: How to Heal with Love, Laughter and Mindfulness*. It's enriched with simple techniques and strategies to optimise wellbeing and enhance positivity when you need it the most.

Working the Laughter Effect

Applying the Laughter Effect in the workplace paves the way for greater creativity, communication and performance. Even if you work from home there are many practices you can integrate into your day to enhance joy.

- **Harness humour in meetings.** Allocate time in your meetings for a lighthearted positive joke or nominate someone to volunteer something funny that happened at home, work or elsewhere. Ensure humour is positive, inclusive and sensitive to diversity.

- **Smile generously and wholeheartedly with your colleagues and clients.** Share your smile on your way to work, at work or on your way home. Start a 'smile squad' in your office – don't laugh. In the early 2000s, police in Victoria enacted a 'Smile Squad' to create a more positive vibe in the neighbourhood.

- **Laughternoon Tea.** Host a laughter-themed lunch session: Laughter Yoga, the science of laughter or smiling and/or laughter meditation.

- **Form a fun committee.** Perhaps the most fun committee ever. A great way to generate giggles and comradery: cook-offs, trivia games, scavenger hunts, an 'anything' tournament, comedy movie break or virtual game night. The list is limitless, as is the laughter potential.

- **Encourage chatter and chortle.** You'll recall the laughter punctuation effect, where most laughter occurs during conversations. (Refer to chapter two.) Create opportunities for informal conversation – potluck lunches where staff bring and share a dish, lunchtime walks or another lunchtime activity.

- **Include icebreakers into teambuilding exercises.** Some activities fit the play and laughter bill perfectly, like 'Two truths and a lie', or 'Who am I?' Or 'Don't laugh', where people go around the circle or progress down a line saying 'ha, ha, ha' until someone bursts into laughter.

- **Random acts of kindness.** Leave a sticky note on a colleague's desk with a smiley face. Buy a co-worker a coffee. Do what you can to make someone's day brighter, especially if it looks like they're having a challenging day. Pay someone a compliment. Leave a yummy treat on a workmate's desk. Wholeheartedly listen to someone's concerns. Share inspiring or humorous memes or quotes.

- **Reframe stressful situations wherever you can with positivity.** Can you find a way to view this specific situation in a different light – to find the funniness or any (remotely) positive outcomes, intended or otherwise? (Please refer to chapter ten for reframing tips.)

- **Make your workplace a grateful space.** Craft a gratitude tree. Leave sticky notes with gestures of thanks and appreciation on colleagues' desks. They can always be anonymous. Write a handwritten note to a colleague – past or present. Say thank you regularly. Create a Wall of Appreciation. (For more ideas on embedding a culture of gratitude see chapter eight.)

- **Speak up the good.** Don't keep positive feedback to yourself, share it with another colleague or their manager.

- **Nominate a Joy Ambassador.** Consider rotating the role monthly to keep things fresh and inspiring.

- **On your way to and/or from work listen to an uplifting or comedic podcast.** A great way to relieve stress and lighten and brighten your mind so you can be more upbeat and present with your co-workers, family and friends.

The Laughter Effect for life

Integrating the Laughter Effect daily has the capacity to transform your life. The more practices you do, the more enlightened you'll become. Create a 'happitat', enriched by humour, laughter and positivity.

- **Tweet or share on social media funny puns or memes.** Create a friends or family What's App group. Join an online group that prioritises humour. There are many to choose from. Share the fun and funny.

- **Attend a Laughter Yoga club – virtually or in person.** There are plenty of options available and online offerings mean you can join any club in the world.

- **Compile a list of funny sitcom series or films to watch later.** Keep your list somewhere accessible so household members can regularly add to it. Ours is on the fridge. Communal viewing will increase the likelihood of laugh-out-loud moments.

- **Create a laughter/humour/play ritual.** What do you love doing that connects you to your inner child and fun-loving version of yourself? Don't leave it to chance – schedule silliness, prioritise play and load up laughter.

- **Humour journal or scrapbook.** Conceptually similar to a gratitude journal but the emphasis is on compiling and collecting things you find funny. Whether that's recounting a funny encounter from your day or looking to cartoons, quotes or memes. On days you need a pick-me-up, flick through your humour stockpile and relive the laughter.

- **Choose a laughter buddy.** A great motivator to ensure your daily dose of laughter. You don't even need to converse; simply choose a time of day and intentionally laugh with each other for a few minutes. Laughter-buddying-up will make you more accountable.

- **Don't leave laughter to chance.** First thing in the morning, laughingly greet yourself in the mirror and choose to laugh outwardly whenever you can. Don't think laughter, laugh laughter.

- **Restore calm in your day with a smile meditation.** The more you connect to your inner smile and fount of wellbeing, the more your inner smile will expand. Regular practice will result in a flow-on effect of genuine and wholehearted smiles throughout the day. (See chapter seven.)

- **Have a news-free day now and again.** The world won't fall apart if you miss a beat, but you might if you don't take a break occasionally. Or try 'cheerscrolling', where you seek out upbeat content – a far brighter option than doomscrolling.

- **Lean into the things and people that make you feel good.** Incorporate mindful moments into your day to notice and reflect on any beneficial sensations, encounters or experiences. Pause and embrace this feel-good energy. The more you pay attention to the micro-moments of goodness in your day, the more goodness you will see.

- **Be kind – to yourself and others – always.** Seek opportunities for random acts of kindness. Not only will the recipient feel better for it, so will you.

- **Restore inner equilibrium by becoming more self-compassionate.** You can't give to others if you've nothing left to give. Tune into your inner talk and note how compassionate or critical it is. (Please refer to chapter nine for self-compassion practices.)

- **Reframe daily stresses with humour or levity.** The stories we tell ourselves can be more emotionally damaging than the event itself. Through journaling or positive reframing we can change our story, revealing a fresh perspective and prospects for greater levity.

- **Grow gratitude.** Demonstrate your appreciation far and wide, not only to your loved ones, but to acquaintances, or people who have provided a service, no matter how small. Handwrite, text or email a note of thank you to someone. Grow goodness in your heart and feel it expand, each day making a mental note or documenting the things and people you are grateful for. Please don't forget yourself in the equation. (Refer to chapter eight for gratitude practices.)

- **Affirm your joy.** Create some affirmations that will turbocharge your wellbeing and joy. Say them out loud or in your head frequently.

- **Elicit your endorphin flow.** Identify your joy source and align your life to it, including as many of these riches in your day as you can. Regularly check in and monitor whether your inner-smile stimuli have changed. Draw on the power of your imagination to further ignite this source. (Please refer to chapter seven for endorphin-boosting practices and how to craft an endorphin board.)

Outline other practices to amplify the Laughter Effect in your life

Glossary

Barrel/bundle of laughs something that's fun or amusing

Belly laugh a loud, deep, uninhibited laugh

Boff a hearty laugh

Cachinnate ('Cack-innate') to lough loudly

Cackle a loud, harsh laugh

Chortle a noisy, gleeful laugh

Chuckle laugh quietly or inwardly

Coulrophobia fear of clowns

Crack up with laughter to laugh with great enthusiasm, or to cause someone to laugh in this way

Gelotology the study of laughter and its effects on the body, from a psychological and physiological perspective

Gelotophilia the joy of being laughed at

Gelotophobia fear of being laughed at

Giggle a light, silly laugh

Giggling Gertie a phrase often used to describe excitable children (FYI there's no male equivalent)

Guffaw laugh loudly and heartily

Homeric laughter an individual laughs loudly and at times uncontrollably for prolonged bouts. The entire body shakes, which is how the gods laughed in Homer's classics

Hoots of laughter a laugh that shows you think something is funny or silly

Howls with laughter a very loud laugh

Laughtershock the feeling of euphoria experienced after an intense amount of laughter. The effects are much like that experienced during and after an adrenalin rush

Roars with laughter to laugh in a noisy way

Shriek with laughter a short and high-pitched laugh

Simper to smile in a silly, affected or ingratiating manner

Snort sudden, intense laugh that exits your body via your nose, causing you to make a humorous sound

Titter to laugh in a nervous or partly suppressed manner

Whoop a loud cry of joy or excitement

> Fun fact: Highest-voted definition of laughter in the Urban Dictionary: 'When a smile has an orgasm.'

ACRONYMS

AIR attention, intention and repetition

BOL burst out laughing

CSL can't stop laughing

FOMCL falling off my chair laughing

LMAO laughing my arse off (or a slightly more polite version: **LMBO** – laugh my butt off)

LMHO laughing my head off

LOL laugh out loud

LOLZ more than one laugh

LOTI laugh on the inside

LQTM laughing quietly to myself

LSHIFOMB laughed so hard I fell off my bed

LSMH laughing and shaking my head

ROFL roll on the floor laughing

SATT smile all the time

SOTI smile on the inside

SOTO smile on the outside

LAUGHTER IDIOMS

Are you having a laugh? are you joking?

For a laugh for fun, for a joke

Good for a laugh fun to be around

Have (someone) laughing in the aisles to cause someone to laugh uproariously and hysterically

Laugh and the whole world laughs with you keep your sense of humour and people will sympathise with you

Laugh a minute very funny (The phrase can also be sarcastically used to describe something that's not funny)

Laughing your head off to be laughing uproariously or hysterically

Laugh till you cry to laugh so hard or intensely that tears come out of one's eyes

Laughing-stock someone who is mocked/ridiculed

No laughing matter something very serious, something that shouldn't be joked about

Piss (oneself) laughing (rude slang) to laugh hysterically or uncontrollably

Play for laughs to do, act or perform with the express intention of being funny

To burst out laughing to laugh suddenly

To have the last laugh to finally be vindicated

To bust a gut to start laughing suddenly or uncontrollably

To die laughing to be overcome with laughter

To laugh all the way to the bank to make a lot of money quickly and easily

To laugh something off to laugh when experiencing something unpleasant to make it seem less serious

To laugh yourself silly to laugh for a long time, to laugh uncontrollably

To split your sides to laugh so hard your body is shaking/convulsing

To have a laugh to joke or kid around; to act or behave in a lighthearted, foolish manner

You've gotta laugh you must try to appreciate that this unfortunate situation is at least a little bit funny

You make me laugh a humorous or sarcastic response to a statement that one thinks is ridiculous or highly improbable, as if it were a joke

Resources

International laughter and humour associations and networks dedicated to happiness, gratitude, self-compassion and optimism:

Action for Happiness (www.actionforhappiness.org)

Association for Applied and Therapeutic Humor: AATH (www.aath.org)

Center for Mindful Self-Compassion (https://centerformsc.org)

Centre for Optimism (www.centreforoptimism.com)

Clowns without Borders (https://clownswithoutborders.org/about-us)

Greater Good Science Center (https://ggsc.berkeley.edu)

International Positive Psychology Association (www.ippanetwork.org)

International Society for Humor Studies: ISHS (www.humorstudies.org)

Laughter Yoga Australia (http://laughteryoga-australia.org)

Laughter Yoga International (https://laughteryoga.org)

Museum of Happiness (www.museumofhappiness.org)

Project Optimism (www.projectoptimism.com.au)

The Home of Laughter Wellness, Laughter Online University (www.laughteronlineuniversity.com)

The Humour Foundation (www.humourfoundation.org.au)

Acknowledgements

Writing this book has been one of my life's greatest pleasures and sharing it with you is a dream.

I owe a debt of gratitude to my husband, Danny, and two gorgeous sons, Josh and Zak, for their abundant love and encouragement. For believing in me and what I do, and supporting my writing journey even when that meant *going troppo* on my quarter gap year. I'm especially grateful to Danny for being my second set of eyes on this book and providing invaluable feedback. To Josh for your creative flair, and Zak for being my personal Deliveroo for all manner of things when I was lost in the flow of writing. My life is immeasurably richer because of all of you.

Thank you to my dear parents, Bridget and Cyril, to whom I dedicate this book, for providing me with opportunities in life to learn and thrive. To my late mother in-law, Lillian, whose love of laughter and pearls of wisdom inspired passages of my writing, and to my late father-in law, Henry, for the many laughter-filled adventures we've shared. Being unconditionally loved and supported by two sets of parents is a blessing indeed.

Wholehearted thanks to my extended family and family of choice for lovingly cheering me on from the sidelines. I am beyond grateful to my posse of best friends for loving me as they do and sustaining me as I ride the waves of life. To my international Laughter Yoga and AATH tribe, it is exhilarating watching you inspire others and spread the laughter ripple. You also win the prize for the most joyous (and riotous) extended family ever.

To my dear friend and laughter colleague Heather Joy Campbell, for early manuscript guidance and input. Thank you for everything. Your middle name personifies the wonderful you.

The Laughter Effect could not have been written without the beautiful souls who have invited me into their private worlds and shared their experiences for others to benefit from. Also, to the many experts and interviewees I spoke with – your wisdom and tales of laughter and life transformation inspired me beyond measure. Researching this book was all the more invigorating owing to the diversity of studies by researchers taking humour and laughter seriously. I can't wait to see what unfolds next!

Serendipity led me to the wonderful Sophy Williams at Black Inc., who enthusiastically embraced my idea for this book from the outset. I'm so grateful for that. To the delightful Kate Morgan for your invaluable editorial feedback and easygoing manner – and to the entire Black Inc. team for your dedication and excitement, which has enabled me to share my mission to spread the Laughter Effect.

And lastly, yet by no means least, to you, dear reader, for choosing this book. May the application of the Laughter Effect promote levity in your life and boost your joy quotient.

About the author

Ros Ben-Moshe is an internationally recognised laughter wellness and positivity expert. She is adjunct lecturer at La Trobe University, where she has taught positive psychology and health promotion. A Global Laughter Ambassador, Ros is a regular commentator and writer in Australian media. Her highly praised first book was *Laughing at cancer: How to Heal with Love, Laughter and Mindfulness.* She has spent over twenty years empowering people to embrace intentional smiling and laughter practices to generate positive life transformation and boost joy.

Notes

CHAPTER 1

1   Mohamed Ben Mansour, 'Laughter in Islam', *Books and Ideas*, https://booksandideas.net/Laughter-in-Islam.html.

2   Warner 1964: 312, in Pearl Duncan, 'The Role of Aboriginal Humour in Cultural Survival and Resistance', PhD thesis, University of Queensland, 2014.

3   Sally L.A. Emmons, 'A Disarming Laughter: The Role Of Humor In Tribal Cultures. An Examination of Humor in Contemporary Native American Literature and Art', University of Oklahoma, 2000, https://shareok.org/bitstream/handle/11244/5983/9975786.PDF?sequence=1&isAllowed=y.

4   Anne Cameron, *Daughters of Copper Woman*, Press Gang Publishers, Vancouver, 1981, p. 109.

5   'Indigenous Games for Children', High Five.org, Ontario, Canada, https://intranet.csf.bc.ca/wp-content/uploads/sites/2/2019/12/ressources/EA_indigenous-games-for-children-en.pdf.

6   Nicole Beaudry, 'Singing, Laughing and Playing: Three Examples from the Inuit, Dene and Yupik Traditions', *The Canadian Journal of Native Studies*, Université du Québec à Montréal, vol. 8. no. 2, 1989.

7   'World's Oldest Joke Traced Back to 1900 BC', Reuters, 1 August 2008, www.reuters.com/article/us-joke-odd-idUSKUA14785120080731.

8   Thomas Fuller, *The History of the Worthies of England*, J. Nichols (ed.), Cambridge Library Collection – British and Irish History, Cambridge University Press, 2015, Doi:10.1017/CBO9781316136270.

9   Denise Selleck, 'On the Trail of Jane the Fool', *On the Issues*, Spring, 1990, www.ontheissuesmagazine.com/1990spring/Spr90_selleck.php.

10 Anna Kelsey-Sugg, 'The Laughing Gas Parties of the 1700s – and How They

Sparked a Medical Breakthrough', *ABC News*, 20 February 2019, www.abc.net.
au/news/2019-02-20/laughing-gas-parties-discovery-of-anaesthesia/10811060.

11   Charles Darwin, C., *The Expression of the Emotions in Man and Animals*, John
Murray, London, 1872, https://doi.org/10.1037/10001-000.

CHAPTER 2

1   Judith Kay Nelson, 'What Made Freud Laugh: An Attachment Perspective on
Laughter', The Sanville Institute for Clinical Social Work and Psychotherapy,
California, USA, 2012, p.16.

2   Caspar Addyman, Charlotte Fogelquist, Lenka Levakova, Sarah Rees, 'Social
Facilitation of Laughter and Smiles in Preschool Children', *Frontiers in
Psychology*, vol. 9, 2018, p.1048.

3   Nelson, 'What Made Freud Laugh' study.

4   Sonja Lyubomirsky, *The How of Happiness: A Scientific Approach to Getting the
Life You Want*, Penguin Press, New York, 2007, p.21.

5   Lea Winerman, 'A Laughing Matter', American Psychological Association, June
2006, https://www.apa.org/monitor/jun06/laughing.

6   Robert Provine, *'The Science of Laughter'*, Psychology Today, 1 November 2000,
https://www.psychologytoday.com/intl/articles/200011/the-science-laughter.

7   Provine, *'The Science of Laughter'*.

8   Karl Grammer and Irenäus Eibl-Eibesfeldt, 'The Ritualisation of Laughter', in
Natürlichkeit der Sprache und der Kultur, Brockmeyer, 1990, pp. 192–214.

9   Grammer and Eibl-Eibesfeldt, 'The Ritualisation of Laughter', pp. 192–214.

10   Kurtz and Algoe, 'Putting Laughter in Context: Shared Laughter as Behavioral
Indicator of Relationship Well-Being', *Journal of the International Association for
Relationship Research*, vol. 22, no. 4, December 2015, pp. 573–90.

11   Laura E. Kurtz and Sara B. Algoe, 'Putting Laughter in Context', pp. 573–90.

12   Doris G. Bazzini, Elizabeth R. Stack, Penny D. Martincin and Carmen P.
Davis, 'The Effect of Reminiscing about Laughter on Relationship Satisfaction',
Motivation and Emotion, vol. 31, no. 1, 2007, pp. 25–34.

13   Freda Gonot-Schoupinsky and Gulcan Garip, 'Prescribing Laughter to Increase
Well-Being in Healthy Adults: An Exploratory Mixed Methods Feasibility Study

of The Laughie', *European Journal of Integrative Medicine*, vol. 26, February 2019, pp. 56–64.

CHAPTER 3

1   'Mental Health-Related Prescriptions', Australian Institute of Health and Welfare, https://www.aihw.gov.au.

2   Norman Cousins, *An Anatomy of an Illness as Perceived by the Patient: Reflections on Healing and Regeneration*, W.W. Norton, New York, 1979, p.43.

3   Thea Zander-Schellenberg, Isabella Collins, Marcel Miché, Camille Guttmann, Roselind Lieb and Karina Wahl, 'Does Laughing Have a Stress-buffering Effect in Daily Life? An Intensive Longitudinal Study', *PLOS One*, vol. 15, no. 7, July 2020.

4   Kei Hayashi, Ichiro Kawachi, Tetsuya Ohira, Katsunori Kondo, Kokoro Shirai, Naoki Kondo, 'Laughter Is the Best Medicine? A Cross-Sectional Study of Cardiovascular Disease Among Older Japanese Adults', *Journal of Epidemiology*, vol. 26, no. 10, October 2016, pp. 546–52.

5   Masao Iwase et al., 'Neural Substrates of Human Facial Expression of Pleasant Emotion Induced by Comic: A PET Study', *Neuroimage*, vol. 17, no. 2, October 2002, pp. 758–68.

6   Mikaela M. Law, Elizabeth A. Broadbent and John J. Sollers, 'A Comparison of the Cardiovascular Effects of Simulated and Spontaneous Laughter', *Complementary Therapies in Medicine*, vol. 37, April 2018, pp. 103–09.

7   Kaori Sakurada et al., 'Associations of Frequency of Laughter with Risk of All-Cause Mortality and Cardiovascular Disease Incidence in a General Population: Findings from the Yamagata Study', *Journal of Epidemiology*, vol. 3, no. 4, April 2020, pp. 188–93.

8   Mary P. Bennett, Janice M. Zeller, Lisa Rosenberg, Judith McCann, 'The Effect of Mirthful Laughter on Stress and Natural Killer Cell Activity', *Alternative Therapies in Health and Medicine*, vol. 9, no. 2, March 2003, pp. 38–45.

9   Lee S. Berk, David L. Felten, Stanley A. Tan, Barry B. Bittman and James Westengard, 'Modulation of Neuroimmune Parameters During the Eustress of Humor-Associated Mirthful Laughter', *Alternative Therapies in Health And Medicine*, vol. 7, no. 2, March 2001, pp. 62–76.

10   Sandra Manninen et al., 'Social Laughter Triggers Endogenous Opioid Release in Humans', *Journal of Neuroscience*, vol. 37, no. 25, June 2017, pp. 6125–31.

11   Adrián Pérez-Aranda et al., 'Laughing Away the Pain: A Narrative Review of Humour, Sense of Humour and Pain', *European Journal of Pain*, vol. 23, no. 2, September 2018, pp. 220–33.

12   Robert I. Dunbar et al., 'Social Laughter Is Correlated with an Elevated Pain Threshold', *Proceedings of the Royal Society of Biological Sciences*, vol. 279, no. 1731, March 2012, pp. 1161–67.

13   Clinton Colmenares, 'No Joke: Study Finds Laughing Can Burn Calories', *Vanderbilt University Medical Center's Weekly Newsletter*, October 2005, https://reporter.newsarchive.vumc.org/index.html?ID=4030.

14   Gurinder Singh Bains et al., 'The Effect of Humor on Short-Term Memory in Older Adults: A New Component for Whole-Person Wellness', *Advances in Mind-Body Medicine*, vol. 28, no. 2, Spring 2014, pp. 16–24.

15   Bernie Warren, 'Spreading Sunshine . . . Down Memory Lane: How Clowns Working in Healthcare Help Promote Recovery and Rekindle Memories'. In N.T. Baum, *'Come to Your Senses: Creating Supportive Environments to Nurture the Sensory Capital Within'*, Toronto, Canada, 2009, pp. 37–44.

16   Lee-Fay Low et al., 'The Sydney Multisite Intervention of LaughterBosses and ElderClowns (SMILE) Study: Cluster Randomised Trial of Humour Therapy in Nursing Homes', *BMJ Open*, vol. 3, no. 1, January 2013.

17   Julie M. Ellis, Ros Ben-Moshe and Karen Teshuva, 'Laughter Yoga Activities for Older People Living in Residential Aged Care Homes: A Feasibility Study', *Australasian Journal on Ageing*, vol. 36, no. 3, July 2017, pp. E28–E31.

18   David Watson, Lee Anna Clark and Auke Tellegen, 'Development and Validation of Brief Measures of Positive and Negative Affect: The PANAS Scales', *Journal of Personality and Social Psychology*, vol. 54, no. 6, 1988, pp. 1063–70.

19   Sonja Lyubomirsky and Heidi S. Lepper, 'A Measure of Subjective Happiness: Preliminary Reliability and Construct Validation', *Social Indicators Research*, vol. 46, no. 2, 1999, pp. 137–55.

20   Rosa Angelo Quintero et al., 'Changes in Depression and Loneliness After Laughter Therapy in Institutionalized Elders', *Biomedica: revista del Instituto Nacional de Salud*, vol. 35, March 2015, pp. 90–100.

21   Mahvash Shahidi et al., 'Laughter Yoga Versus Group Exercise Program in Elderly Depressed Women: A Randomized Controlled Trial', *International Journal of Geriatric Psychiatry*, vol. 26, no. 3, year to come, pp 322–27.

22   Mohammad Reza Armat, Amir Emami Zeydi et al., 'The Impact of Laughter Yoga on Depression and Anxiety Among Retired Women: A Randomized Controlled Clinical Trial', *Journal of Women & Aging*, vol. 26, no. 3, March 2011, pp. 322–27.

23   C. Natalie van der Wal and Robin N. Kok, 'Laughter-Inducing Therapies: Systematic Review and Meta-Analysis', *Social Science & Medicine*, vol. 232, July 2019, pp. 473–88.

24   Paul N. Bennett, Trisha Parsons, Ros Ben-Moshe et al., 'Intradialytic Laughter Yoga Therapy for Haemodialysis Patients: A Pre-post Intervention Feasibility Study', *BMC Complementary and Alternative Medicine*, vol. 15, article no. 176, June 2015.

25   So-Hee Kim et al., 'The Effect of Laughter Therapy on Depression, Anxiety, and Stress in Patients with Breast Cancer Undergoing Radiotherapy', *Journal of Korean Oncology Nursing*, vol. 9, no. 2, August 2009, pp. 155–62.

26   Tahmine Tavakoli et al., 'Comparison of Laughter Yoga and Anti-Anxiety Medication on Anxiety and Gastrointestinal Symptoms of Patients with Irritable Bowel Syndrome', *Middle East Journal of Digestive Diseases*, vol. 11, no. 4, October 2019, pp. 211–17.

27   Takashi Hayashi et al., 'Laughter Up-regulates the Genes Related to NK Cell Activity in Diabetes', *Biomedical Research*, vol. 28, no. 6, 2007, pp. 281–85.

28   Shevach Friedler et al., 'The Effect of Medical Clowning on Pregnancy Rates After In Vitro Fertilization and Embryo Transfer', *Fertility and Sterility*, vol. 95, no. 6, May 2011, pp. 2127–30.

29   Jocelyn Lowinger, 'Laughter Plays Tricks with Your Eyes', ABC Science online, 3 February 2005, https://www.abc.net.au/science/news/health/HealthRepublish_1294404.htm.

30   Anthony Rivas, '"Mirthful" Laughter Keeps Memory Loss at Bay, Benefits the Brain as Much as Meditation', *Medical Daily*, 28 April 2014, https://www.medicaldaily.com/mirthful-laughter-keeps-memory-loss-bay-benefits-brain-much-meditation-279254.

31   Nairán Ramírez-Esparza et al., 'No Laughing Matter: Latinas' High Quality of Conversations Relate to Behavioral Laughter', *PLOS ONE*, vol. 14, no. 4, article e0214117, April 2019.

32 Yudai Tamada et al., 'Does Laughter Predict Onset of Functional Disability and Mortality Among Older Japanese Adults?', *Journal of Epidemiology*, vol. 31, no. 5, 2021, pp. 301–07.

33 H. Kimata, A. Morita, S. Furuhata et al., 'Assessment of Laughter by Diaphragm Electromyogram', Eur J Clin Invest 2009, vol. 39, no. 1, pp. 78–9, in Ramon Mora-Ripoll, 'Potential Health Benefits of Simulated Laughter: A Narrative Review of the Literature and Recommendations for Future Research', *Complementary Therapies in Medicine*, vol. 19, no. 3, June 2011, pp. 170–77.

34 Dexter Louie, Karolina Brook and Elizabeth Frates, 'The Laughter Prescription: A Tool for Lifestyle Medicine', *American Journal of Lifestyle Medicine*, vol. 10, no. 4, September 2014, pp. 262–67.

CHAPTER 4

1 Statistics from the government of Mexico City, Undersecretary of Penitentiary System, https://penitenciario.cdmx.gob.mx/poblacion-penitenciaria, obtained in May 2022.

CHAPTER 5

1 Sigmund Freud, *The International Journal of Psycho-Analysis*, vol. 9, London, 1928, in 'Humor and Life Stress: Antidote to Adversity', Herbert M. Lefcourt and Rod A. Martin, Springer-Verlag, 1st edition, 1986.

2 Liane Gabora and Kirsty Kitto, 'Toward a Quantum Theory of Humor', *Frontiers in Physics*, vol. 4, no. 53, January 2017.

3 Steven M. Sultanoff, 'Levity Defies Gravity, Using Humor in Crisis Situations', *Therapeutic Humor*, vol. 9, no. 3, Summer 1995, pp. 1–2.

4 'Laughter May Be Best Medicine for Brain Surgery: Effects of Electrical Stimulation of Cingulum Bundle', *Science Daily*, 4 February 2019, https://www.sciencedaily.com/releases/2019/02/190204170932.htm.

5 Norman Cousins, *Head First: The Biology of Hope*, E.P. Dutton, New York, 1989, p. 126.

6 Rod A. Martin et al., 'Individual Differences in Uses of Humor and Their Relation to Psychological Well-being: Development of the Humor Styles Questionnaire', *Journal of Research in Personality*, vol. 37, no. 1, 2003, pp. 48–75.

7   William Larry Ventis, Garrett Higbee and Susan A. Murdock, 'Using Humor in Systematic Desensitization to Reduce Fear', *Journal of General Psychology*, vol. 128, no. 2, 2001, pp. 241–53.

8   VIA Survey of Character Strengths, Positive Psychology Center, University of Pennsylvania, https://ppc.sas.upenn.edu/resources/questionnaires-researchers/survey-character-strengths.

9   Liliane Müller & Willibald Ruch, 'Humor and Strengths of Character', *The Journal of Positive Psychology*, vol. 6, 2011, pp. 368–76.

10   Chaya Ostrower, *It Kept Us Alive: Humor in the Holocaust*, Yad Vashem, Israel, 2014, p.60.

11   Ostrower, *It Kept Us Alive: Humor in the Holocaust*.

12   Wesley A. Kort, 'review of *Redeeming Laughter: The Comic Dimension of Human Experience* by Peter L. Berger', in *Theology Today*, vol. 56, no. 1, pp. 134–36.

13   Barbara L. Fredrickson, 'The Role of Positive Emotions in Positive Psychology: The Broaden-And-Build Theory of Positive Emotions', *The American Psychologist*, vol. 56, no. 3, March 2001, pp. 218–26.

14   Hilde M. Buiting et al., 'Humour and Laughing In Patients with Prolonged Incurable Cancer: An Ethnographic Study in a Comprehensive Cancer Centre', *Quality of Life Research: An International Journal of Quality of Life Aspects of Treatment, Care and Rehabilitation*, vol. 29, no. 99, April 2020, pp. 2425–34.

15   Hilde M. Buiting et al., 'Humour and Laughing In Patients with Prolonged Incurable Cancer: An Ethnographic Study in a Comprehensive Cancer Centre', pp. 2425–34.

16   Steven M. Sultanoff, 'Levity Defies Gravity: Using Humor to Help Those Experiencing Crisis Situations', *Therapeutic Humor*, vol. 9, no. 3, Summer 1995, pp. 1–2.

17   Robert Half, 'Is a Sense of Humour in the Workplace Good for Your Career?', Robert Half Talent Solutions, 27 March 2017, https://www.roberthalf.com.au/blog/jobseekers/sense-humour-workplace-good-your-career.

18   'Bell Leadership Study Finds Humor Gives Leaders the Edge', Business Wire, 20 March 2012, https://www.businesswire.com/news/home/20120320005971/en/Bell-Leadership-Study-Finds-Humor-Gives-Leaders-the-Edge.

19 Jennifer Aaker and Naomi Bagdanos, 'How to Be Funny at Work', *Harvard Business Review,* 5 February 2021, https://hbr.org/2021/02/how-to-be-funny-at-work.

20 Karen O'Quin and Joel Aronoff, 'Humor as a Technique of Social Influence', *Social Psychology Quarterly,* vol. 44, 1981, pp. 349–57.

21 Brian Daniel Vivona, 'Humor Functions within Crime Scene Investigations: Group Dynamics, Stress, and the Negotiation of Emotions', *Police Quarterly,* vol. 17, no. 2, May 2014, pp. 127–49.

22 Jelena Brcic et al., 'Humor as a Coping Strategy in Spaceflight', *Acta Astronautica,* vol. 152, November 2018, pp. 175–78.

23 Joe A. Cox, Raymond L. Read and Philip M. Van Auken, 'Male–Female Differences in Communicating Job-related Humor: An Exploratory Study', *Humor,* vol. 3, no. 3, 1990, pp. 287–96.

24 Eiman Azim et al., 'Sex Differences in Brain Activation Elicited by Humor', *Proceedings of the National Academy of Sciences of the United States of America,* vol. 102, no. 45, November 2005, pp. 16496–501.

CHAPTER 6

1 Sigmund Freud, *Jokes and Their Relation to the Unconscious,* W.W. Norton, New York, 1963, p. 15.

2 Judith Kay Nelson, *What Made Freud Laugh – An Attachment Perspective on Laughter,* Routledge, New York, 2012.

3 Mary Beard, 'A History of Laughter – From Cicero to *The Simpsons*', *The Guardian,* 28 June 2014, https://www.theguardian.com/books/2014/jun/28/history-laughter-roman-jokes-mary-beard.

4 Sigmund Freud, *Jokes and Their Relation to the Unconscious,* p. 137.

5 Peter Derks et al., 'Laughter and Electroencephalographic Activity', *Humor: International Journal of Humor Research,* vol. 10, no. 3, 1997, pp. 285–300.

6 P. Shammi and Donald Thomas Stuss, 'Humour Appreciation: A Role of the Right Frontal Lobe', *Brain,* vol. 122, no. 4, April 1999, pp. 657–66.

7 Paul E. McGhee, *Health, Healing and the Amuse System: Humor as Survival Training,* Kendall/Hunt Publishers, Iowa, 1999.

8   Ken Makovsky, 'Behind the Southwest Airlines Culture', 21 November 2013. https://www.forbes.com/sites/kenmakovsky/2013/11/21/behind-the-southwest-airlines-culture/?sh=2664c4263798.

9   Kristin Robertson, 'Southwest Airlines Reveals 5 Culture Lessons', Human Synergists International, 24 June 2022, https://www.humansynergistics.com/blog/culture-university/details/culture-university/2018/05/29/southwest-airlines-reveals-5-culture-lessons.

10 'Why Workplace Humour is the Secret to Great Leadership', Rise, 23 October 2018, https://risepeople.com/blog/why-workplace-humour-is-the-secret-to-great-leadership/.

11 Mindful Staff, 'Why Vulnerability Is Your Superpower', 20 November 2018, https://www.mindful.org/why-vulnerability-is-your-superpower/.

12 J.L.Teslow, 'Humor Me: A Call for Research', Educ Technol Res Dev vol. 43, pp. 6–28, 1995 in Brandon M. Savage, Heidi L. Lujan, Raghavendar R. Thipparthi, Stephen E. DiCarlo, 'Humor, Laughter, Learning, and Health! A Brief Review', Advances in Physiology Education, vol. 41, no. 3, July 2017, pp. 341–47.

13 Brandon M. Savage et al., 'Humor, Laughter, Learning, and Health! A Brief Review', pp. 341–47.

14 Kazunori Nakanishi, 'Using Humor in the Treatment of an Adolescent Girl with Mutism: A Case from Japan', Psychoanalysis, Self and Context, vol. 12, no. 4, September 2017, pp. 367–76.

15 Magda Szubanski, Reckoning: A Memoir, Text Publishing, Melbourne, 2015.

16 Lisa Wagner, 'The Social Life of Class Clowns: Class Clown Behavior Is Associated with More Friends, but Also More Aggressive Behavior in the Classroom', Frontiers in Psychology, vol. 10, no. 604, April 2019.

17 The UN Refugee Agency, https://www.unhcr.org/refugee-statistics.

18 Jaak Panksepp and Jeff Burgdorf, '"Laughing" Rats and the Evolutionary Antecedents of Human Joy?', Physiology & Behavior, vol. 79, no. 3, August 2003, pp. 533–47.

19 Elise Wattendorf et al., 'Exploration of the Neural Correlates of Ticklish Laughter by Functional Magnetic Resonance Imaging', Cerebral Cortex, vol. 23, no. 6, April 2012, pp. 1280–89.

20 Dacher Keltner and George A. Bonanno, 'A Study of Laughter and Dissociation:

Distinct Correlates of Laughter and Smiling During Bereavement', *Journal of Personality and Social Psychology*, vol. 73, no. 4, 1997, pp. 687–702.

CHAPTER 7

1   Barbara Wild et al., 'Neural Correlates of Laughter and Humour', *Brain,* vol. 126, no. 10, October 2003, pp. 2121–38.

2   Guillaume-Benjamin-Amand Duchenne de Bologne, *Mechanism of Human Facial Expression: Studies in Emotion and Social Interaction*, Cambridge University Press, 1990, p. 31.

3   Mark G. Frank, Paul Ekman and Wallace V. Friesen, 'Behavioral Markers and Recognizability of the Smile of Enjoyment', *Journal of Personality and Social Psychology*, vol. 64, no. 1, 1993, pp. 83–93.

4   The Newsroom, 'One Smile Can Make You Feel a Million Dollars', *The Scotsman*, 4 March 2005, https://www.scotsman.com/health/one-smile-can-make-you-feel-million-dollars-2469850.

5   Alicia A. Grandey et al., 'Is "Service with a Smile" Enough? Authenticity of Positive Displays During Service Encounters', *Organizational Behavior and Human Decision Processes*, vol. 96, no. 1, January 2005, pp. 38–55.

6   Andreas Hennenlotter et al., 'The Link Between Facial Feedback and Neural Activity within Central Circuitries of Emotion: New Insights from Botulinum Toxin-Induced Denervation of Frown Muscles', *Cerebral Cortex*, vol. 19, no. 3, March 2009, pp. 537–42.

7   Sven Söderkvist, Kajsa Ohlén and Ulf Dimberg, 'How the Experience of Emotion Is Modulated by Facial Feedback', *Journal of Nonverbal Behavior*, vol. 42, no. 1, September 2017, pp. 129–51.

8   Ernest L. Abel and Michael L. Kruger, 'Smile Intensity in Photographs Predicts Longevity', *Psychological Science*, vol. 21, no. 4, February 2010, pp. 542–44.

9   LeeAnne Harker and Dacher Keltner, 'Expressions of Positive Emotion in Women's College Yearbook Pictures and Their Relationship to Personality and Life Outcomes Across Adulthood', *Journal of Personality and Social Psychology*, vol. 80, no. 1, 2001, pp. 112–24.

10   Matthew J. Hertenstein et al., 'Smile Intensity in Photographs Predicts Divorce Later in Life', *Motivation and Emotion*, vol. 33, no. 2, June 2009, pp. 99–05.

11 Barbara L. Fredrickson and Marcial F. Losada, 'Positive Affect and the Complex Dynamics of Human Flourishing', *American Psychologist*, vol. 60, no. 7, October 2005, pp. 678–86.

12 'First Impressions Are Everything: New Study Confirms People with Straight Teeth Are Perceived as More Successful, Smarter and Having More Dates', Cision PR Newswire, 19 April 2012, https://www.prnewswire.com/news-releases/first-impressions-are-everything-new-study-confirms-people-with-straight-teeth-are-perceived-as-more-successful-smarter-and-having-more-dates-148073735.html.

13 Fritz Strack, Leonard L. Martin and Sabine Stepper, 'Inhibiting and Facilitating Conditions of the Human Smile: A Nonobtrusive Test of the Facial Feedback Hypothesis', *Journal of Personality and Social Psychology*, vol. 54, no. 5, 1988, pp. 768–77.

14 Tom Noah, Yaacov Schul and Ruth Mayo, 'When Both the Original Study and Its Failed Replication Are Correct: Feeling Observed Eliminates the Facial-Feedback Effect', *Journal of Personality and Social Psychology*, vol. 114, no. 5, May 2018, pp. 657–64.

15 Tara L. Kraft and Sarah D. Pressman, 'Grin and Bear It: The Influence of Manipulated Facial Expression on the Stress Response', *Psychological Science*, vol. 23, no. 11, September 2012, pp. 1372–78.

16 Sven Söderkvist, Kajsa Ohlén and Ulf Dimberg, 'How the Experience of Emotion Is Modulated by Facial Feedback', *Journal of Nonverbal Behavior*, vol. 42, no. 1, September 2017, pp. 129–51.

17 William Bloom, *The Endorphin Effect: A Breakthrough Strategy for Holistic Health and Spiritual Wellbeing*, Piatkus, London, 2011, p. 28.

CHAPTER 8

1 Rick Hanson, *Hardwiring Happiness: The New Brain Science of Contentment, Calm, and Confidence*, Harmony Books, New York, 2013.

2 Martin E.P. Seligman et al., 'Positive Psychology Progress: Empirical Validation of Interventions', *American Psychologist*, vol. 60, no. 5, July–August 2005, pp. 410–21.

3 Leah Dickens and David DeSteno, 'The Grateful Are Patient: Heightened Daily Gratitude Is Associated with Attenuated Temporal Discounting', *Emotion*, vol. 16, no. 4, June 2016, pp. 421–25.

4   Paul J. Mills, 'A Grateful Heart Is a Healthier Heart', American Psychological Association, 6 April 2015, http://www.apa.org/news/press/releases/2015/04/grateful-heart.

5   Asif Amin et al., 'Gratitude & Self esteem Among College Students, *Journal of Psychology & Clinical Psychiatry*, vol. 9, no. 4, July 2018.

6   Summer Allen, 'The Science of Gratitude', Greater Good Science Center, May 2018, https://www.templeton.org/wp-content/uploads/2018/05/GGSC-JTF-White-Paper-Gratitude-FINAL.pdf.

7   Sheung-Tak Cheng, Pui Ki Tsui and John H.M. Lam, 'Improving Mental Health in Health Care Practitioners: Randomized Controlled Trial of a Gratitude Intervention', *Journal of Consulting and Clinical Psychology*, vol. 83, no. 1, pp. 177–86.

8   Christine Porath and Douglas R. Conant, 'The Key to Campbell Soup's Turnaround? Civility', *Harvard Business Review*, 5 October 2017, https://hbr.org/2017/10/the-key-to-campbell-soups-turnaround-civility.

9   Douglas R. Conant, 'Secrets of Positive Feedback', *Harvard Business Review*, 16 February 2011, https://hbr.org/2011/02/secrets-of-positive-feedback.

10   Kristin D. Neff, Kristen L. Kirkpatrick and Stephanie S. Rude, 'Self-compassion and Adaptive Psychological Functioning', *Journal of Research in Personality*, vol.41, no.1, February 2007, pp. 139–154.

CHAPTER 9

1   Marcella Raffaelli & Lenna L. Ontai, 'Gender Socialization in Latino/a Families: Results from Two Retrospective Studies', Sex Roles, vol. 50, 2004, pp. 287–99, in Lisa M. Yarnell et al. : 'Meta-Analysis of Gender Differences in Self-Compassion, Self and Identity', vol. 14, no. 5, 2015, pp. 499–520.

2   Joachim Stoeber, Alexandra Feast and Jennifer Hayward, 'Self-oriented and Socially Prescribed Perfectionism: Differential Relationships with Intrinsic and Extrinsic Motivation and Test Anxiety', Personality and Individual Differences, vol. 47, 2009, pp. 423–28.

3   Paul L. Hewitt et al., 'The Multidimensional Perfectionism Scale: Reliability, Validity and Psychometric Properties in Psychiatric Samples', *Psychological Assessment*, vol. 3, no. 3, 1991, pp. 464–68.

4   Juliana G. Breines and Sarina Chen, 'Self-compassion Increases

Self-improvement Motivation', *Personality and Social Psychology Bulletin*, vol. 38, no. 9, September 2012, pp. 1133–43.

5   Neff and Vonk, 'Self-compassion Versus Global Self-esteem: Two Different Ways of Relating to Oneself', pp. 23–50.

6   Jia Wei Zhang et al., 'A Compassionate Self Is a True Self? Self-Compassion Promotes Subjective Authenticity', *Personality and Social Psychology Bulletin*, 2019, https://self-compassion.org/wp-content/uploads/2019/08/ZhangJW_etal2019.pdf.

7   Kristin D. Neff and Andrew P. Costigan, 'Self-Compassion, Wellbeing and Compassion', *Psychologie in Österreich*, vol. 2, 2014, pp. 114–19.

8   Serena Chen, 'Give Yourself a Break – The Power of Self Compassion', *Harvard Business Review*, Sept–Oct 2018, https://hbr.org/2018/09/give-yourself-a-break-the-power-of-self-compassion.

9   Tara Brach, *Radical Compassion: Learning to Love Yourself and Your World with the Practice of RAIN*, Ebury Publishing, London, 2020.

CHAPTER 10

1   Leda Cosmides, John Tooby, 'Evolutionary Psychology and the Emotions', *Handbook of Emotions*, 2000, in Michael A. Cohn et al., 'Happiness Unpacked: Positive Emotions Increase Life Satisfaction by Building Resilience', *Emotion*, vol. 9, no. 3, June 2009, pp. 361–68.